International Case Studies in Mental Health

EDITORS

Senel Poyrazli
The Pennsylvania State University

Chalmer E. Thompson
Indiana University–Purdue University Indianapolis

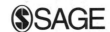

SAGE

Los Angeles | London | New Delhi
Singapore | Washington DC

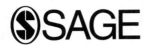

Los Angeles | London | New Delhi
Singapore | Washington DC

FOR INFORMATION:

SAGE Publications, Inc.
2455 Teller Road
Thousand Oaks, California 91320
E-mail: order@sagepub.com

SAGE Publications Ltd.
1 Oliver's Yard
55 City Road
London, EC1Y 1SP
United Kingdom

SAGE Publications India Pvt. Ltd.
B 1/I 1 Mohan Cooperative Industrial Area
Mathura Road, New Delhi 110 044
India

SAGE Publications Asia-Pacific Pte. Ltd.
3 Church Street
#10-04 Samsung Hub
Singapore 049483

Acquisitions Editor: Kassie Graves
Editorial Assistant: Courtney Munz
Production Editor: Cassandra Margaret Seibel
Copy Editor: Michelle Ponce
Typesetter: Hurix Systems Private Ltd.
Proofreader: Rae-Ann Goodwin
Indexer: Terri Corry
Cover Designer: Candice Harman
Marketing Manager: Terra Schultz
Permissions Editor: Adele Hutchinson

Printed in the United States of America

A catalog record of this book is available from the
Library of Congress.

ISBN 978-1-4129-9035-6

This book is printed on acid-free paper.

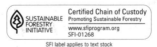

Certified Chain of Custody
SUSTAINABLE FORESTRY INITIATIVE
Promoting Sustainable Forestry
www.sfiprogram.org
SFI-01268
SFI label applies to text stock

12 13 14 15 16 10 9 8 7 6 5 4 3 2 1

International Case Studies in Mental Health

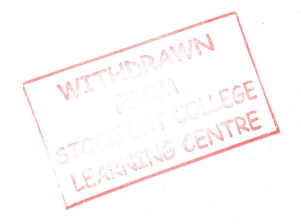

Contents

Foreword

Modernism has produced remarkable advances in the science and practice of psychology. The modernist perspective is grounded in logical positivism: investigative approaches that separate the person from the intertwined conditions in which he or she is situated and the linear interpretation of objective measurements of basic psychological structures and processes. Modernism has its limitations, however. It has become increasingly clear that the tenets and methods of a modernist psychology are not universally applicable but instead reflect the ecological milieu in which this variant of the discipline thrived. Very likely, this realization has been influenced by globalization, which has made explicit a new reality comprised of many diverse psychologies, including U.S. psychology. All psychologies have distinctive as well as common features, each of which expresses a larger worldview shaped by culture, economics, history, politics, religion, and, of course, the individual.

Globalization can be seen in the increased worldwide movement of capital as well as goods and services, the rise of representative forms of government and concern with human rights, growth in the transnational migration of large numbers of peoples, and the explosive exchange of information through digital communication technologies. Irrespective of its benefits and costs, globalization has led to innovative adaptations to an ever more interconnected and interdependent world. The speed and extensiveness of globalization, and its psychosocial and sociocultural consequences, have challenged psychologists to review the implicit assumptions on which their theories, research, and applied practices rest. This critical examination has energized alternative disciplinary perspectives and movements, such as multiculturalism and indigenization, which offer a counterweight to the modernist paradigm. Such developments have been a clarion call for greater multilateral, horizontal dialogue among psychologists in the industrialized and majority (developing) worlds. Such dialogue has enriched the conceptual, empirical, and applied knowledge and skills of all psychologists in their efforts to understand more fully and respond more effectively to the nuanced domains in which human beings live.

The *Universal Declaration of Principles for Psychologists* was conceived as common moral framework that would inspire and guide psychologists worldwide toward the highest ethical ideals in their professional activities. The four principles of the *Universal Declaration* are Respect for the Dignity of Persons and Peoples, Competent Caring for the Well-Being of Persons and Peoples, Integrity, and Professional and Scientific Responsibilities to Society. These principles are especially relevant for the growing number of counselors, psychotherapists, and healers who often are tasked to work with highly diverse and underserved indigenous and immigrant, refugee, or sojourner populations in their home countries or abroad. Ethical practice mandates not only that practitioners do no harm but also that they endeavor to improve quality of life by offering contextually appropriate services to individuals, couples, families, groups, communities, and society as a whole. Thus, problems in living and psychological dysfunction need to be viewed as the local expression of symptoms found in either universal or culture-bound disorders or as an adjustment to oppressive circumstances (e.g., poverty, violence). Western taxonomies like the *Diagnostic and Statistical Manual of Mental Disorders* may need to be augmented by locally meaningful representations of mental illness. Procedurally, practitioners need to respect local customs and weigh the advantages and risks of introducing folk remedies, community healers, and normative styles of relating to their standard treatment repertoire.

Paradoxically, while practitioners are expected to provide ethically unimpeachable and evidence-based interventions domestically and internationally, there frequently is a wide gulf between the idealized depictions and the stark realities of treatment that can leave practitioners confused, frustrated, and hesitant to work with clients and in settings where their talents are sorely needed. Practitioners may find themselves hand-tied as they strain to improve lives if equipped with didactic and experiential learning that is frozen in a monocultural and monolingual status quo or that falls prey to simplistic exhortations to assess a host of client demographics and explore overgeneralized group differences. Psychology associations, professional training programs, faculty instructors and clinical supervisors, and organizers of continuing education are at a crossroads: The demand for effective multicultural and international interventions requires that curricular materials and pedagogical techniques evolve to ensure the preparation of full-capacity global citizens, a necessary precondition for context-centered, ethical engagement by current and future practitioners. One unmistakable response to the challenge just noted is this book: *International Case Studies in Mental Health*.

In *International Case Studies in Mental Health*, Senel Poyrazli and Chalmer E. Thompson designed a unique chapter template that introduces the reader to the rich detail with which to situate each case study. After summarizing the background and treatment orientation of the chapter authors and featured practitioner, the cultural and sociopolitical conditions of the country from which the case was drawn are highlighted, along with local perspectives on mental health problems, mental healthcare, and mental health providers. Relevant life-history data, selected client variables, presenting concerns, and a case conceptualization are described; followed by the form, process, and course of treatment; and concluding with an evaluation of its successful outcomes and unresolved issues. Several chapters provide guidelines for working appropriately and effectively in similar circumstances, particularly suggestions for harnessing community resources to enhance the viability and impact of intervention. The authors and practitioners, who often partnered internationally on each chapter, are acknowledged experts in counseling, psychotherapy, and healing and represent industrialized and majority countries from the six inhabited continents, including the United States. The case studies range from problems in living to occasionally debilitating psychopathology and are written so masterfully that they invariably evoke the strengths and limitations of the client and practitioner and the humanity of their therapeutic collaboration. Poyrazli and Thompson also include introductory and concluding chapters that orient the reader to the case study format and integrate significant thematic material across case studies.

There is much to learn from *International Case Studies in Mental Health,* whether the reader is a graduate student, clinical supervisor, faculty instructor in a professional training program, or a mental health practitioner interested in or currently working with diverse and underserved populations domestically or abroad. Among the recurrent themes of the volume are the synthesis of diverse yet complementary frameworks for treatment (e.g., contextual action theory, multicultural case conceptualization); the fusing of modernist approaches with indigenous procedures and religious and social customs (e.g., Mayan cosmology, *curanderismo,* and the Catholic mass in Guatemala); the importance of the personal and reputational qualities of the practitioner that serve to mitigate cultural mistrust and permit accurate understanding of symptoms (e.g., headaches, eccentric thinking); the co-creation of a working relationship unencumbered by biased assumptions via inclusive cultural empathy (i.e., balancing client and practitioner similarities and differences and understanding the treatment relationship in its cultural context); the empowerment of clients by strengthening mindfulness and protective factors and by improving psychological and social harmony; the expanded definition of the helper role to include the support functions of culture broker and advocate when building needed community linkages; the assessment of multiple acculturative stressors and acculturative strategy when working with immigrants, refugees, and sojourners; and caution not to overgeneralize from a single case study given the demographic and sociocultural heterogeneity found within groups.

Psychology has a social responsibility to address the needs and facilitate the aspirations of the world's peoples. For psychology to become more responsive, it must undertake with imagination and vigor the increasingly urgent challenge of becoming more attuned to diverse cultural and socio-political worldviews without abandoning entirely the modernist theories, research methods, and applied practices that have enriched our understanding of human functioning and experience. One heartening response to this challenge is the emergence of international psychology, a field whose mission is to increase the frequency, broaden the scope, and enhance the meaningfulness of communication and collaboration among psychologists and psychology students with shared interests from diverse countries and cultures via curriculum, scholarship, advocacy, and networking. Without a doubt, *International Case Studies in Mental Health* advances the mission of international psychology. It is a groundbreaking volume, which given its relevance and timeliness, will only gain in stature.

Michael J. Stevens, PhD, DHC
Illinois State University, United States
The Lucian Blaga University, Romania

Preface

This book presents a variety of cases from around the world. The people described within these pages—the ones who seek help to eliminate their distress and those who provide the help—come from both developed and developing countries. In most of the cases, the helpers share a similar heritage with the help seekers and are influenced at least partly by Western psychotherapy traditions. The treasure to behold in these cases is the authors' strivings: Academic psychologists and practitioners collaborate to describe the confluence of cultural and sociopolitical influences that tailor the treatment and in so doing, inform a pathway to effective healing. Each chapter is a showcase of how psychologists and mental health practitioners worldwide collaborate to achieve invaluable work.

Our purpose in writing this book is to help prepare both mental health trainees and practicing professionals to be effective in the provision of healing in their work with people in different regions of the world. Consequently, we hope to offer practitioners a glimpse of what can be achieved in these regions by people whose reputations within the respective communities are strong. Far from representing what occurs in each and every case, we instead attempt to provide details about these contexts, about the particular skills and mindsets of the practitioners, and details of the people in search of psychic relief. Moreover, with increases in migration, sojourning, and the disappearance of borders, we believe this book responds to the call of many university training program leaders who want to expand their curriculum to include cases from countries outside of their own.

We wanted to create a volume that stands out from others in important ways. To date, there have been no books devoted entirely to describing cases from an international perspective. This book therefore fills a void in the field. Furthermore, rather than examining case studies that include individuals from outside of the United States to the exclusion of U.S. cases, we accomplish both. We believe this feature of inclusion reflects our desire to resist a practice of *othering* in cultural psychology, that is, of subtly conveying that the United States is the rightful purveyor of countries outside of itself. In addition, readers of the volume learn not only of the cases themselves but also about different contextual conditions that may affect an individual's mental health functioning. The work of mental health practitioners in each chapter shows how different factors (racial-ethnic culture, gender, age, sexual orientation, religion and spirituality, socioeconomic status, sociopolitical conditions, etc.) contribute to an individual's functioning. Each chapter shows how these factors may influence the counseling and psychotherapy relationship between the client or patient and the mental health practitioner.

We envision this book will benefit a variety of different groups and can be used in many contexts:

- This book benefits students in the mental health professions and particularly those who intend to work abroad or with immigrant populations.
- This book benefits mental health practitioners who are already working in the field in broadening their scope of practice.
- The book can be used as a main textbook in graduate internship seminars.
- The book can be used as a companion book in required courses in multiculturalism, such as multicultural competency, cross-cultural counseling, or cross-cultural therapy.

We would like to acknowledge the contribution and help many individuals provided that led to this book coming to fruition: the authors of the chapters; editors and assistants at SAGE Publications, particularly Ms. Kassie Graves; and many friends and family members who motivated us and provided encouragement.

Introduction

Toward an Inclusive International Psychology

Senel Poyrazli, PhD
Chalmer E. Thompson, PhD

Culture colors every aspect of human existence. It presents us with an unspoken guide for determining what is important and how we are to relate to one other and conduct our lives. It includes assumptions about stratified hierarchies in a society, like race, the expected roles of men and women, the manner in which authority figures are heeded, and the sociopolitical structures that order our lives in ways we may not always be aware. Yet another aspect of culture, one that emerges most clearly from the multitude of books written on the topic, is that it is learned (Mukhoopadhyay, Henze, & Moses, 2007). No one is born with a particular culture.

Indigenous approaches to helping people alleviate the stressors of life, reduce debilitating symptoms, and cope with trauma and grief also are learned. These approaches can be handed down from past generations. The timeworn, yet essential, facets that are most associated with psychic healing are maintained, even after thousands of years as with African psychology (Nobles, 1972; Parham, 2009), and metamorphisized to best suit the needs of the contemporary generation. Even with Western hegemony, those influences that come from the United States and Europe that are transported to other nations, cause mental health practice throughout the world to become nuanced, and bring forth the best of what wealthier nations can offer combined with the best of what developing nations can offer. From the powerful influence of Western culture, we have scientific research that tests approaches and a wealth of scholarship that guides the training of professionals. From developing nations we have generations-long traditions of helping as well as communal rituals and mores that acknowledge the connection of the individual with the broader whole.

The main purpose of this book is to feature the counseling and therapeutic work of mental health practitioners and thus illustrate how highly recognized healers have learned as cultural beings to conceptualize, intervene, and evaluate the effectiveness of their practices with the people who need their help. These revered practitioners are from all over the world; both helper and help seeker alike, in most cases, come from the same region of the world. Although there are indigenous approaches included in the collection of cases, the vast majority of our practitioners make use of a variety of approaches, selecting the best of what they've learned from mostly traditional psychology training programs and devising their own ways of effectively helping the help seekers. Notably, each chapter situates the practitioner and help seeker within a cultural context. Our contributors present rich descriptions of culture, race, and other sociocultural or sociopolitical forces that shape the people in the respective regions and influence the practitioners' assessment and intervention. Our goal is to deepen the readers' understanding of how the cultural context influences client functioning and by extension, practitioner and client interactions. Therefore, we view our collection as a sort of world stage in which mental health intervention is played and where our audience can capture the meaning of sage Martín-Baró's (1994) words, in his book *Writings for a Liberation Psychology,* that psychology is not and can never be seen as being removed from history and context, and that all proclivities to commit such erasures deeply affect everyone who is a member of the particular society. Cushman (1995) agrees, cautioning practitioners who believe that the distillment of Western approaches can viably be exported to other countries, he wrote:

> Nothing has cured the human race, and nothing is about to. Mental ills don't work that way; they are not universal, they are local. Every era has a particular configuration of self, illness, healer, technology; they are a kind of cultural package. They are interrelated, intertwined, interpenetrating. So when we study a particular illness, we are also studying the conditions that shape and define that illness, and the sociopolitical impact of those who are responsible for healing it. (p. 7)

Fundamental to each of the case studies is how both practitioner and client come to ascribe meaning to what constitutes adequate or optimal functioning within that society.

Our uses of the terms *mental health* and *healing* or *healer* are deliberately broad to recognize the variations that exist in the practitioner's terminology particular to their society. We also requested that our contributors label the terms they normally use to refer to the people they treat.

As two international psychologists, we believe that as psychology continues to expand beyond borders, it is vital that we educate would-be practitioners about the resources that already exist in different regions of the world. Moreover, we have a profound appreciation of multicultural psychology, which paved the way for the more recent cross-national psychology (Heppner et al., 2009). Emerging out of the civil rights movement of the 1950s and 1960s, multicultural psychology has a scholarship that examines acculturation, racial and ethnic identity, cross-racial and ethnic discourse in psychotherapy process, cultural equivalence in intelligence and personality assessment, and so on (see Shea & Leong, this volume; Heppner et al., 2009). More importantly, multicultural psychology historically has urged practitioners to examine the contextual forces that give shape to psychological functioning and development—a clear outcry against a U.S. hegemony that has committed physical and psychological violence against people of color (Guthrie, 1998). The thrust of multicultural psychology is to inform and widen understanding of the lifeways, perspectives, and humanity of all people in a manner that is respectful and caring. It is on the pillars of this psychology which we stand. Hence, what we strive to do within these pages is to advance the best of what international psychology has to offer. The goal of international psychology is "to promote communication and collaboration among psychologists worldwide" so that the field of psychology around the world can further develop (Stevens & Wedding, 2004, p. 1). We hope that our book contributes to what international psychology tries to achieve and illustrates how great collaborations among psychologists worldwide can be accomplished.

Our book also contributes to internationalizing the psychology curriculum efforts. In recent years, many organizations, researchers, and instructors have emphasized the importance of internationalizing the psychology curriculum and showed efforts towards accomplishing this goal. For example, the American Psychological Association's (APA) Division of International Psychology (Division 52) formed a curriculum and training committee to gather and disseminate information about how faculty members internationalize their courses (Grenwald, n.d.). In addition, many textbook authors either wrote new books related to international psychology or updated their existing books to include international content (e.g., Brock, 2009; Denmark, Krauss, Wesner, Midlarsky, & Gielen, 2005; Feldman, 2010; Gerstein, Heppner, Aegisdottir, Leung, & Norsworthy 2009; Gibbons & Stiles, 2004; Malley-Morrison & Hines, 2003; Pickren & Rutherford, 2010; Stevens & Wedding, 2004). These efforts helped the field of psychology to move from "western psychology is universal" to "there are different psychological knowledge bases in every country and culture."

When we selected the authors for our chapters, we proceeded very carefully. We wanted to have international psychologists who were noted and senior psychologists who were actively engaged within their professional organizations and who participated in teaching, service, or research activities in other countries. These psychologists were invited to write a chapter by identifying a prominent mental health practitioner in the country from which the case would come. We also instructed all authors to follow research ethics, seek permission from their institutional review boards for research, and follow proper consent procedures for the case. We also shared with the authors our vision for this book and the fact that we wanted the cases to be discussed based on multiculturalism (e.g., Hays, 2007). The authors were to include in their chapters how different factors (race-ethnicity, gender, age, sexual orientation, socioeconomic status, religion and spirituality, etc.) played a role in the client's or patient's mental health and how the very same factors may have influenced the therapeutic relationship between the client or patient and the mental health practitioner. We invited a diverse group of authors and attempted as best we could to include a balance of male and female clients. Our authors have made ample use of references by scholars from their own countries and, specifically, from those who can address the particularities of their clients' distresses. Our striving is to combat the marginalization that too often characterizes the field of psychology with respect to how problems are understood, defined, and treated.

The Chapters

Each chapter presented in this book provides an introduction of the authors, detailed information about the practitioner, contextual conditions of the country from which the case came, the presenting problem of the client or patient, the treatment provided, and an evaluation of the treatment. Some chapters also provide suggestions for treating similar clients or patients.

In Chapter 1, Ladislav Valach and Richard Young describe Switzerland's sociocultural and political landscape, as they also share details of their case of Mrs. Kirchberg, a 45-year-old woman who seeks professional help from the first author. As her therapist, Dr. Valach employs mainly cognitive behavioral strategies to help his patient resolve the distress that keeps her from pursuing constructive life goals. Her pursuit of these goals was dramatically hampered after discovering how seriously ill her brother had become and that she, following a pattern in her family, was expected to assume much of his care. Mrs. Kirchberg finds herself emotionally out of sorts, feeling as though she will fail her brother, herself, and her family, and she lacks the energy to accomplish virtually any task. Using contextual action theory as an integrative framework for organizing, planning, and executing therapy interventions, Dr. Valach helps Mrs. Kirchberg by creating and maintaining a solid working alliance throughout the therapy, which is ongoing, intervenes in timely ways to provide the fullest benefit of the treatment plan, and ensures that in-therapy learning is extended to the patient's life outside of therapy. A richly detailed chapter with multiple sources for readers to consult for further information about the framework, the authors reveal how characteristics of the therapist, combined with an arsenal of well-timed and well-executed skills, result in desirable outcomes for the patient.

The case from Sierra Leone is presented by Ani Kalayjian and Georgiana Sofletea (Chapter 2). The authors describe a very moving story of a child-soldier who was a victim and a perpetrator at the same time. The atrocities described in the chapter and the initiation process the client went through when he was recruited by the Militia are overwhelming. The authors tell of the client's escape from the Militia, his daily struggle to survive as he hid in the forest with other children who also escaped the Militia, and how he came out from hiding when the civil war ended. The client, 24 years of age at the time, received a two-day group treatment, individual face-to-face sessions, and individual phone-session treatments that were based on the Seven-Step Biopsychosocial and Eco-Spiritual Model created by Dr. Kalayjian. The treatment was provided through an organization that Dr. Kalayjian founded. The mission of the organization is to provide a range of outreach activities to people around the world who are affected by natural- and human-created disasters. The treatment the client received was part of the outreach effort to alleviate trauma in former child soldiers and individuals with physical disabilities. The chapter describes how the client was guided in ways of forgiving himself, in finding how to deal with the exclusion he experienced by members of his community, and in pursuing an educational and career path to help him integrate into the society.

Sexual abuse of children, crisis intervention, and advocacy work are portrayed in the chapter from Zimbabwe (Chapter 3). Becoming aware of and then facing children—very young children—who have been sexually abused is an experience so difficult to fathom that not all practitioners are able to take on such cases. Dr. Margaret Rukuni feels she has no other option as child sexual abuse has increased in her native Zimbabwe in the past several years. Like too many instances in which communities are tragically affected by extreme poverty, conflict, and neglect by the world's superpowers as children and families go hungry, there is an unraveling of families and of extended kinships. Dr. Rukuni recounts her therapy work with two children traumatized by repeated sexual abuse by a once-trusted young boy who is the son of the family's landlady. The shock of the news does not result in an immediate removal of the children; the family is at first immobilized, in conflict with each other, and dare we say, afraid of the monetary gains they'll lose in changing their place of residence. Dr. Rukuni is no less jarred by the ugly and bizarre features of this case. She talks of her own needs for restoration. In acting as an advocate for the young girls, she accompanies the family to the court, a system that is not a friend to the victims of abuse.

The practitioner's description of her work, together with Dr. Thompson and Rev. Ajabu's brief description of Zimbabwe's sociopolitical backdrop, gives readers a snapshot of the extent of dedication and skill necessary to help children and families overcome the adversities of violence, the fallibility of parents and parent figures amidst a distressed society, and the significance of assuming two roles, that of therapist and advocate.

In Chapter 4, the case study from Turkey, written by Senel Poyrazli and Mehmet Eskin, the authors point out important cultural and religious consequences to the decision to come out and behave openly as a nonheterosexual person. In this chapter, a bisexual man's attempt to reject his identity as a result of discrimination towards lesbian, gay, bisexual, and transgendered (LGBT) groups present both in law and practice in a Turkish context is described and how this attempt leads to severe psychosomatic symptoms is presented. The client's difficulty resisting the demands of his family as well as resisting the societal expectation that he get married to a woman is described. Dr. Eskin uses a combination of a person-centered approach and cognitive behavioral therapy to help the client eliminate his psychosomatic symptoms and accept his bisexuality. The chapter also discusses some positive developments within the country to help reduce negative attitudes and prejudice towards LGBT persons. The authors of the chapter suggest that for clients who are from a more collectivistic and traditional culture as compared to some of the Western cultures, an approach where the client is helped to find ways to balance his or her needs and goals with cultural expectations will likely lead to a more effective treatment outcome and better mental health for the client.

Our only case from the Arab world comes from Lebanon (Chapter 5). Brigitte Khoury shares the case of a middle-aged woman who is stuck between her own family and her parents. This is a unique case in that it illustrates how the needs of nuclear families can be in conflict with the cultural norms of the extended families to be involved in the nuclear family's affairs. When this conflict is not resolved, it can lead to depression and anxiety just like the case illustrates. Khoury presents a culturally balanced treatment model that helps the patient in this case to find a balance between inserting her individual right to have more freedom related to her own nuclear family, while at the same time attending to the social needs of her parents. Working with Systems Theory, Khoury helps the patient understand how power differences within the extended family likely contribute to the patient's depression and anxiety. Khoury also helps the patient see that while it is important to keep the social support that comes from closeness in the family relationships, culturally appropriate insertion of individual rights is also important, especially if this closeness leads to negative emotions and experiences, causing the individual to have psychological symptoms. Khoury demonstrates that the key to providing successful treatment in Lebanese culture is to find a way to balance between the nuclear family's need for a certain level of independence and the nuclear family's cultural obligation and allegiance to its families of origin.

In Chapter 6, the case selected by Changming Duan, Xiaoming Jia, and Yujia Lei draws vivid attention to how the counselor's attention to cultural context factors can be interwoven in a (relatively) nondirective therapy with a Chinese client. The authors describe the case of a young male college student whose academic successes, although the foci of praise and family glory, have contributed paradoxically to the client's feelings of isolation and depression. Balancing psychodynamic and person-centered theories, the counselor and supervisor in the case address the significance of familial piety and other cultural qualities that inform their assessment and treatment of the client. Dr. Jia, one of the pioneers of counseling in China, supervises this case with Lei as the counselor. The description of how supervisor and counselor talk about the dynamics that occur within the counseling, including the counselor's feelings about the client's boastfulness and, at one point in the therapy, working through the client's awkward revelations about his sexual desires, help illustrate important topics for future learning on psychotherapeutic care. The authors also note the recent surge of Westernized counseling practices on college campuses throughout the world's most populous country. The authors present wise discussions of how China's modernization in recent years can emerge into greater tendencies toward individualism and the potential costs of this change to the mental health of current-day and future China.

In Chapter 7, Lawrence H. Gerstein, Young Soon Kim, and TaeSun Kim present the treatment of a female Korean client based on the Han Counseling Model, an indigenous model in Korea. The chapter describes therapist Young Soon's search for a counseling model that better fits the Korean culture than Western models. Her search led to the Han Counseling Model which is based on Han ideology. In this ideology, humans are the most important beings; they are a part of the heaven, earth, and universe. By using this indigenous counseling model, Young Soon provides treatment to a middle-aged female client who is having difficulty balancing several roles, experiencing marital conflict, and having problems with her son. The case in this chapter illustrates how, with modernization, women in Korea have more pressure to be nurturing mothers as well as effective workers. In the chapter, we see that the therapist's work with Han counseling creatively intertwines Korean thinking with modern issues to provide mental health treatment. The authors of the chapter point readers' attention to moving away from a Eurocentric perspective of treatment to instead creating and using culturally appropriate models.

Andrés J. Consoli, María de los Ángeles Hernández Tzaquitzal, and Andrea González describe the treatment of a Guatemalan teenager in Chapter 8. At the beginning of the chapter, they critically examine the marginalization of indigenous people throughout Guatemalan history, but also point readers' attention to some positive developments in the country towards valuing ethnic and cultural diversity. The authors inform readers about mental health services in the country as well as social injustices in the distribution of governmental funding for these services, with more funds going to urban settings, resulting in further marginalization of indigenous groups who tend to live in the rural areas. The authors describe the customs of the Mayans, one indigenous group in Guatemala, and how this group relies primarily on spirituality as a means to cope with mental health problems. The case described in the chapter is related to a 17-year-old Mayan female adolescent. She experiences some psychotic symptoms that are based on her spiritual beliefs. The extreme stress she is under leads to her seeing a light in her room, feeling the presence of images and figures, and feeling the pressure of a hand around her neck. In the chapter, we also see the therapist's skillful case conceptualization and the integration of her Western training with her knowledge of Mayan spiritual beliefs to carry out successful treatment. At the end of the chapter, the authors present important suggestions for mental health practitioners working with Mayan individuals.

Disaster Shakti is an organization that responds to people who face the brutal consequences of human and natural disasters—the devastating spread of AIDS in villages leaving unprecedented numbers of children without parents; the horrific physical damage, governmental neglect, and violence targeted to the mostly impoverished residents of Ward 6, New Orleans following Hurricanes Katrina and Rita; and the focus of this chapter, the considerable loss in lives, physical structures, and services in an already beleaguered Haiti in the aftermath of the January 12, 2010 earthquake. Author Gargi Roysircar, in Chapter 9, writes about the needs of a psychological approach to disaster response that is not pathologically based, that is not confined to one or a set of theories (she frames these as "theories wars"), and which fundamentally is ecologically in its reach. Also essential to disaster response is the expertise of mental health providers who can recognize shock and trauma symptoms as well as signs of depression, especially when the residents of the setting may not deem these symptoms as such. But perhaps more important than merely identifying those outward symptoms that signal psychological distress, Dr. Roysircar and her team of students apply the best of what mental health practitioners provide. They recognize what is needed, how to work with others who come to assist in the disaster response, and how to help build on the coping reserves that already exist. How important indeed would it be for those who come to assist the already beleaguered not to exclusively heap on charity but instead to expertly wield all manner of intervention to get to the heart of the problem, capitalize on the strengths of cultural traditions, and take every care to be respectful of world views that may counter those of their own? Dr. Roysircar shares a composite case of a Haitian family whose mother is terminally ill with stomach cancer and who has suffered a bevy of recent tragedies that threaten family stability. In this composite case, the father of the family is killed from the collapse of a building during the earthquake. The belief that one of the daughter's husbands willed this disaster poses a welcome challenge to Roysircar as she helps the family over the course of a long day.

At the outset, Clay and Thompson note in Chapter 10 that Black men in the United States are among the populations whose images in print and electronic media are painted ominously negatively. As two Black women psychologists who are from the Washington, DC, area and who have close relationships with Black men, Clay and Thompson chime in to recognize the conundrums that can exist between Black men and women and the bombardment of societal messages that can pit them against the other (White & Peretz, 2010). Dr. Clay describes Mr. T, a 59-year-old Black man whose foray into counseling began with a focus on how he wanted to work to overcome his depression and sense of isolation and estrangement from his wife and children. Dr. Clay was inspired by M. Maultsby, a Black psychologist, who developed Rational Behavioral Therapy. Dr. Clay presents with actual raw data from her assessment of Mr. T and reveals how the use of client homework is helpful in relieving his depression and sense of isolation.

In our final international case study, Chapter 11, Shea and Leong situate their case description of Mr. P. and his treatment within the Cultural Accommodation Model (CAM) of psychotherapy (Leong & Lee, 2006). The authors illustrate how the use of the CAM can help guide practitioners in incorporating traditional models of psychotherapy with the yields of a burgeoning multicultural literature to develop culturally sensitive case conceptualizations and treatments. Dr. Shea's client, Mr. P., is a 47-year-old Chinese man who grew up in Hanoi in 1960—in the midst of the very violent, oppressive, and intractable Vietnam War—who presents with auditory hallucinations, grandiose thinking, and other severe psychiatric symptoms. In a chapter that begins with personal revelations about her own experiences as a Chinese woman who immigrated to the United States as a student, Dr. Shea reveals how she eventually became professionally invested in learning how different experiences of immigration have an impact on individual immigrants and notably, how best to help these special clients or patients through the process in her role as psychologist. The author provides a captivating account of how she collaborates with Mr. P. to best discern his needs and the roots of some of his complaints. She also exposes how the hospital staff at Mr. P.'s facility often hastily made decisions about his care based on racial and ethnic generalizations, leading to a failure to probe more fully into the contours of his complaints. The authors discuss the importance of the role of advocacy for patients in settings and provide an example of how there may be a tendency for some hospital staff to medicate patients when they have somatic complaints, rather than probe more carefully and sensitively into their complaints.

In conclusion, we strongly believe that this book is a needed addition to the mental health literature around the world because in it we attempt to show how knowledge about culture, inclusive of sociopolitical issues, ultimately is what we need to improve psychological theory, research, and practice. We believe that this book contributes to the goal of international psychology by giving an opportunity to mental health practitioners from different parts of the world to collaborate and demonstrate that great work can be accomplished through this collaboration. These collaborations are built on mutual respect, certainly a key feature to building solidarity. Each partnership also acknowledges the strengths of a people as well as the challenges that keep the collective from prospering spiritually, socially, and economically. We hope that the readers of this book benefit from the work of our authors as a result of reading the chapters, increasing their knowledge related to different mental health practices around the world, and finding ways to incorporate this knowledge into their research, teaching, consultation, or clinical practice.

References

Brock, A. (2009). *Internationalizing the history of psychology*. New York: NYU Press.

Cushman, P. (1995). *Constructing the self, constructing America: A cultural history of psychotherapy*. Reading, PA: Addison-Wesley.

Denmark, F. L., Krauss, H. H., Wesner, R. W., Midlarsky, E., & Gielen, U. P. (Eds.). (2005). *Violence in the schools: A cross-cultural and cross-national perspective*. New York, NY: Springer.

Feldman, R. S. (2010). *Adolescence*. Upper Saddle River, NY: Prentice Hall.

Gerstein, L. H., Heppner, P. P., AEgisdottir, S., Leung, S-M. A., & Norsworthy, K. L. (2009). *International handbook of cross-cultural counseling: Cultural assumptions and practices worldwide*. Thousand Oaks, CA: Sage.

Gibbons, J. L., & Stiles, D. A. (2004). *Thoughts of youth: An international perspective on adolescents' ideal persons*. Greenwich, CT: Information Age.

Grenwald, G. (n.d.). Curriculum and training committee: Online survey on internationalizing psychology courses [Web log post]. Retrieved from http://www.internationalpsycology.net

Guthrie, R. V. (1998). *Even the rat was white: A historical view of psychology* (2nd ed.). Needham Heights, MA: Allyn & Bacon.

Hays, P. A. (2007). *Addressing cultural complexities in practice, assessment, diagnosis, and therapy*. Washington, DC: American Psychological Association.

Heppner, P. P., AEgisdottir, S., Seung-ming, A. L., Duan, C., Helms, J. E., Gerstein, L. H., & Pederson, P. B. (2009). The intersection of multicultural and cross-national movements in the United States: A complementary role to promote culturally sensitive research, training, and practice. In L. H. Gerstein, P. P. Heppner, S. AEgisdottir, Leung, S. A., & Norsworthy, K. L (Eds.). *International handbook of cross-cultural counseling: Cultural assumptions and practices worldwide* (pp. 33–52). Thousand Oaks, CA: Sage.

Leong, F. T. L., & Lee, S. H. (2006). A Cultural accommodation model of psychotherapy: Illustrated with the case of Asian-Americans. *Psychotherapy: Theory, Research, Practice, and Training, 43*, 410–423.

Malley-Morrison, K., & Hines, D. (2003). *Family violence in a cultural perspective: Defining, understanding, and combating abuse.* Thousand Oaks, CA: Sage.

Martín-Baró, I. (1994). *Writings for a liberation psychology.* Cambridge, MA: Harvard University.

Mukhopadhyay, C. C., Henze, R., & Moses, Y. T. (2007). *How real is race? A sourcebook on race, culture, and biology.* Lanham, MD: Rowman & Littlefield Education.

Nobles, W. W. (1972). African philosophy as a foundation for Black psychology. In R. L. Jones (Ed.). *Black Psychology* (pp. 18–32). New York, NY: Harper & Row.

Parham, T. A. (2009). Foundations for an African American psychology. In H. A. Neville, B. M. Tynes, & S. O. Utsey (Eds.). *Handbook of African American psychology* (pp. 3–18). Thousand Oaks, CA: Sage.

Pickren, W., & Rutherford, A. (2010). *A history of modern psychology in context.* New York, NY: Wiley.

Stevens, M. J., & Wedding, D. (2004). International psychology: An overview. In M. J. Stevens & D. Wedding (Eds.). *Handbook of international psychology* (pp. 1–21), New York, NY: Brunner-Routledge.

White, A. M., & Peretz, T. (2010). Emotions and redefining Black masculinity movements of two profeminist organizers. *Men and Masculinities, 12*, 403–424.

1

The Case Study of Therapy With a Swiss Woman

An Action Theory Perspective

Ladislav Valach
Richard A. Young

The following case is presented by Richard Young and Ladislav Valach, who

_____ **Introduction of the Authors**

The following case is presented by Richard Young and Ladislav Valach, who
have known each other and worked together for more than 20 years. Valach,
a psychologist and psychotherapist in private practice in Switzerland,
provided the treatment of this patient. As a licensed psychotherapist in
Switzerland, he successfully completed the requisite clinical training and has
practiced as a psychotherapist since 1998. Valach also engaged in an extensive university teaching and research career in psychology at the Universities
of Bern and Zurich as well as at an outpatient clinic of a university hospital. Thus, he is considered effective and known for providing professional
practice in psychology in his community. Young is a professor of counseling
psychology at the University of British Columbia and is a registered psychologist in British Columbia. Valach and Young worked jointly in elaborating
what has come to be known as contextual action theory (Valach, Young, &
Lynam, 2002; Young, Valach, & Collin, 1996, 2002; Young et al., 2011).
This perspective has both an associated research method and implications
for practice.

The Practitioner

Valach is seen as an effective psychotherapist for several reasons. His training, during which he was supervised by well-regarded clinicians, prepared him for the kind of work described in this chapter. From our experiences, the results of Dr. Valach's work with patients are seen as effective by our colleagues, the physicians and psychiatrists with whom we work. His supervisor has reported a high level of satisfaction with Dr. Valach's work in terms of theoretical adherence.

Finally, the patients themselves, as gleaned from their own reports to Dr. Valach at the conclusion of therapy, suggest that the issues for which they sought therapy are no longer present and they are able to go on with their lives, engaging in the required and desired actions, projects, and careers. Valach practices within cognitive-behavioral therapy in general and in cognitive-behavioral therapy with an interpersonal focus in particular (Grawe, 2004). He integrates various approaches within this frame of reference into the broader view of the contextual action theory approach that is discussed in this chapter.

The words *patient, therapist,* and *therapy* are used routinely in this chapter. While the distinction between counseling and psychotherapy can be drawn on the basis of whether the individuals presenting themselves for treatment have a diagnosed mental illness, our view is that there is greater overlap than difference between psychotherapy and counseling as practices. Indeed, both therapy and counseling have to be able to address issues arising from unconscious processes and emotional memory as well as those arising in everyday life. To do less is to short circuit treatment. Our choice of using the terms *patient, therapist,* and *therapy* in this chapter is influenced by the location of the treatment. Valach's practice is situated in a medical context. Thus, these terms are commonly used.

The Case

The patient is a woman in her early forties, married with three children in their late teens, and is small in stature with short hair and a sporty appearance. For the purposes of this chapter, she is identified as Mrs. Kirchberg, a fictitious name. Following the custom of professional relationships in Switzerland, the therapist addressed her as Mrs. Kirchberg and she addressed the therapist as Dr. Valach. He did not address her by her first name. Mrs. Kirchberg agreed and signed an agreement for the use of her narrative as well as the description of the patient-therapist encounters in this chapter.

In the first session, Mrs. Kirchberg complained that she suffered because of lack of energy since her brother's emergency hospitalization during which he was in coma. During this experience, her parents showed complete helplessness in organizing the treatment of their son and the necessary formalities connected to his matters, and Mrs. Kirchberg felt alone. When asked about it, she identified a similar feeling at the time of early puberty when her parents argued a lot, initially separated, and then reunited. During this period, Mrs. Kirchberg protected and supported her mother and her mother's point of view in the family arguments. But, in the end, she had to give in when her mother decided to return to her husband. Mrs. Kirchberg's father was impulsive and had a violent temper. She was afraid of him, although he seldom hit her. Her father accused his wife of infidelity, and Mrs. Kirchberg only learned many years after the accusation that her mother had an extramarital affair. She indicated that had she known this, she would have not sided with her mother, based on the reasoning of her innocence. When Mrs. Kirchberg found out the truth, she felt very helpless and at the mercy of others.

Mrs. Kirchberg was very moved when she spoke about missing being acknowledged and recognized by her father and about her self-esteem. She also described another time, four years ago, when she felt very weak. Her then 15-year-old daughter became depressed after she had been excluded from her soccer team. Mrs. Kirchberg further mentioned her 10-year-long engagement in community politics and how she left because of the antagonistic atmosphere. She had begun her political involvement when her children started their schooling.

Mrs. Kirchberg mentioned that she never wanted to burden her children with her problems as her mother did to her sister. Mrs. Kirchberg complained about her relationship with her sister who has divorced twice, and married a man who, as she put it "never worked and had no money." Mrs. Kirchberg's sister constantly asked Mrs. Kirchberg for financial support. This relationship is addressed toward the end of the treatment when Mrs. Kirchberg intensified her contact with her sister for occupational reasons. Mrs. Kirchberg complained about intrusive and recurrent thoughts. In this chapter we concentrate on only two facets of Mrs. Kirchberg's case: the family of origin issue and Mrs. Kirchberg's relationship challenges with her daughter. The issue with the patient's husband and her vocational issues as they are related to these two issues are mentioned only briefly.

The Context

Switzerland is a sophisticated Western European country with a well-developed educational and health system. Citizens expect professionals to have appropriate qualifications and to be monitored by the appropriate professional bodies. It is customary for psychological services to be offered by professionals, although like many countries, there is a range of services offered by nonprofessionals. Users of professional services assume the effectiveness of these services based on the credentials of the service provider and, ultimately, on a scientific worldview.

Relative to this case, the therapist is a competent health care provider specializing in psychology and credentialed in psychotherapy. He has added legitimacy because he practices within a medical context (the other three colleagues in the practice community are medical doctors), and the costs of his services are covered by the health insurance that is compulsory for all inhabitants of Switzerland (because he works in an arrangement called delegation in which the psychiatrist takes the responsibility for the treatment and bills the patient). Thus, this service is utilized by all classes, and the majority of patients are referred to psychotherapy by their family physician. Nevertheless, some groups of the population utilize these services more than others, such as females more than males, middle-aged people more than young people, immigrants more than those born in the country, and so on.

One of the most relevant long-term contextual aspects of the case of this female patient is the development of the situation of women in Swiss society in the last 100 years. Switzerland became industrialized later than some other European countries, such as France, Great Britain, and Germany. Further, due to the stable social situation during the first half of the 20th century, Switzerland did not experience any rapid social and demographic changes as did some other European countries, for example, the mobilization of many women for industry during World Wars I and II. Thus, the transformation from traditional to modern social roles for women in Switzerland took a longer time than in many other industrialized European countries. This delay in transformation was not only in political rights (voting was introduced at the federal level in 1972) but also in the expectation that women should not take up education and jobs outside their homes, the patriarchal family organization, and women's self-understanding of their role in the family and in relationships. At the same time, the divorce rate rose; for example, between 1984 and 2009, it increased from 28.9 to 47.7 per 100 marriages (Federal Statistical Office, 2011a). In addition, people in Switzerland, perhaps because of having neither a royal court nor a strong centralized government with an extensive administration, adhere more to practical work and working experience than to academic education required for jobs in civil service. Thus, being successful in the occupational world is seldom tied to seeking higher education. This is seen more so in women, as less middle-aged and older women possess higher education or training than men, although the young women nowadays often represent a majority in higher education (particularly in nontechnical disciplines). During the 2008 to 2009 school year, the tertiary education system had 234,799 students (49.7% female). While the proportion of females in obligatory schools remained unchanged between 1980 and 2010, at about 48.6%, the proportion of females attending universities rose by more than 50% from 32.5% in 1980 to 50.1% in 2010. This is relevant for the patient in this case, as she became qualified attending apprenticeship without higher education.

Also relevant for this therapy is the situation of foreign-born citizens in Switzerland, as the therapist is identified as one of them, although he has been living in Switzerland since 1969. Switzerland experienced a large immigration in the last 50 years. In the last 10 to 20 years, a substantial part of the population distanced itself from immigrants for two distinct reasons (Gross, 2006). One group of immigrants, often from the Balkan area and Turkey, is largely composed of unqualified workers, of whom the younger often circulate in groups in public places and display hostile and violent behavior. The second large immigrant group is composed of well-qualified people, mostly from Germany, who, coming from a different educational system, possess school and university diplomas the Swiss citizens might not have and who, consequently, compete for the qualified jobs (Müller-Jentsch, 2008). In 2009, 30% of the foreign population between the age of 25 and 64 had no post compulsory school education or training (only about 13% of the Swiss had no post compulsory school education or training), but about 30% of the foreign population between 25 and 64 possessed a tertiary education (30% of the Swiss had a tertiary education, but only due to the introduction of universities of applied sciences in 1997 which helped raise the number of tertiary educated from 22% in 1996 to 35% in 2010) (Federal Statistical Office, 2011b).

Further, the patient, though not particularly religious, comes from a frugal, work-oriented Protestant culture, in which achievement and maintaining a low profile are high values, while the therapist grew up in the Catholic, visual, and baroque cultural tradition of the former Czechoslovakia. As far as social stratification and social class system is concerned, Switzerland is, apart from certain part of the foreign population, a fairly homogenous society, though not in wealth but in social lifestyle. So, despite all these social differences between the patient and the psychotherapist their everyday life is somehow similar because of the lifestyle homogeneity of the Swiss society.

Of further relevance are substantial changes in the educational system in Switzerland in the last 15 years in which many universities of applied sciences opened, offering a broad range of various courses for people without the classical university entrance eligibility education. Until recently the institutions of education and schooling, political participation and taking up political office, compulsory military service, and civil defense were the "melting pot" where all people met and engaged in common purposes without class or wealth barriers. Flaunting upper class manners is widely unpopular in Switzerland even among affluent classes. However, some recent trends may challenge the homogeneity of the Swiss society. Only recently private schools started booming, offering a better education to the affluent. Military service, the traditional integrative institution of people from the three language cultures of Switzerland, became less popular and relevant as a career facilitator. The relevance of civil defense, another integrative and classless institution, declined. Due to the increased mass media role in politics, language eloquence, speed of thinking, and photogenity became selection criteria for politicians with the consequence that the professional classes suddenly became overrepresented in the political institutions. Nevertheless, until recently the education standard was an apprenticeship (over 60% of the population) providing a basis for the homogeneity of this society.

The Treatment

Mrs. Kirchberg was seen 27 times (and continues in therapy) in the course of one year, for a 90-minute session on each occasion. This is not unusual for dealing with the problems this patient presented. The 90-minute sessions are the therapist's choice backed up by the health insurance. Her narrative in the first session, presented in the previous section, is the presenting problem. In that session, the therapist encouraged Mrs. Kirchberg to tell her narrative, confirming her identity goals (that is, how the patient wants to be seen) and helping her to engage with her emotions (Michel & Valach, 2010). Feelings and emotional expression were invited, for example, missing being recognized by her father and about her self-esteem. A secure frame for these expressions was provided and the search for similar emotional experiences encouraged. The patient and therapist discussed relaxation exercises (patient was familiar with autogenous training, a relaxation technique devised in the first half of the last century by J. H. Schultz [1937]) and performed a counting and breathing exercise. "Thinking aloud" of thoughts and feeling was the initial help provided to deal with intrusive thoughts. Some *projects* established early in her life such as "I have to be responsible for the family happiness and peace," and adopted as a lifelong *career,* were identified. These italicized terms are explained in a later section. The therapist also explained the formal psychotherapy procedures (health insurance and so forth). Following her first utterances, the patient was assured that the therapist understood her Swiss-German dialect well, though he did not speak it.

Evaluation of the Treatment

This series of therapy sessions between Mrs. Kirchberg and the therapist is discussed from the perspective of contextual action theory, although the therapist primarily used other therapeutic modalities. Thus, the well-known principles and techniques of the cognitive-behavioral therapy will be not elaborated upon. Contextual action theory was applied by the therapist as an integrative framework to understand both the therapy process and parallel experiences in the patient's life. It is used by therapists and counselors for this purpose. Briefly, contextual action theory is based on the premise that people understand their own and others' behavior as goal directed (Young, Valach, & Collin, 1996, 2002). When actions coalesce as having a common goal over a midterm length of time, they are identified as a project. In this case, the therapy itself can be understood as a joint project between the therapist and Mrs. Kirchberg. Grouping projects together over a long time period contribute to the construction of career. For example, in this case, the patient's relationship career is evident from her narrative. Actions, projects, and careers are steered by socially shared goals. They are controlled and regulated by internal thoughts and feelings and by the communication between participants in joint actions and projects. They are also constituted by specific behaviors reflective of skills, habits, unconscious processes, and internal and external resources.

Young and colleagues (Young et al., 2011) identified the following five primary therapeutic tasks from an action-theory perspective: (1) creating and maintaining a working alliance, (2) helping the client link therapy and life processes, (3) helping the client identify systems and levels of projects and actions, (4) helping the client to deal with emotion and emotional memory, and (5) helping the client search for optimal goals, strategies, and regulation processes in his or her relevant ongoing processes. These tasks are the basis for the following discussion of this case.

Creating and Maintaining the Working Alliance

One of the most important tasks in psychotherapy is creating and maintaining the working alliance (Constantino, Castonguay, & Schut, 2002; Michel & Jobes, 2011). The client-counselor relationship is critical to successful outcomes (Martin, Garske, & Davis, 2000). It is characterized by genuineness and authenticity, and the intentionality of both participants is recognized. Thus, the working alliance becomes an important paradigm for understanding and acting on the relationship in therapy as well as providing an important model for goal-directed processes generally. Once in a relationship, therapy and higher order skills, such as counselor self-awareness and paying attention to how particular situations or challenges are handled, apply.

Establishing the working alliance and relationship is the first issue in the client-counselor/psychotherapist encounter, and it remains the highest priority throughout therapy. So from the first moment of the therapist's encounter with Mrs. Kirchberg, all the therapist's actions were guided by the goal of achieving a good working alliance. However, we suggest that therapists should simultaneously be aware of and engaged in the other four tasks also identified above. This enables the therapist to understand the context of therapy and the principles behind these processes as well as the aims of the client/therapist joint work, before being fully able to pursue and develop a working alliance. Thus, therapists and counselors are able to build their working relationship together with the client/patient based on the personal experiences and action system of the client.

We distinguish two sources for building a working alliance. The first attempt to establish a working alliance is anchored in the general cultural rules and conventions of politeness, manners, empathy, customer-related skills, and the like. These conventions are important. Polite, friendly, empathic conduct; a friendly, tasteful, clean, and inviting environment; clear and simple language; and observance of the conventional rules of conduct in this culture help establish a good relationship. These rules imply a correct but friendly, and neither too formal nor too relaxed, greeting and invitation. An attentive inquiry, brief and never overly verbose interventions, and keeping a low profile are parts of these conventions. We do not underestimate the power of first impressions in everyday life obtained in the first seconds of an encounter. Of course, counselors and psychotherapists can be particularly skilled in connecting with the client in these first moments, but there is much more to the working alliance than a friendly encounter. Building up a working alliance is not limited to a few strategies used in the first session. Rather, it is the constant work during the whole of therapy. Thus, it must be well integrated in the understanding of ongoing processes. That is, it must be a part of the systemic joint action order of the goal-directed processes. The therapist engages in the patient's current ongoing, goal-directed systems or rather in those that they set up together in order to support these patient's facilitative goal-directed processes. In doing this, the therapist can then balance the various goals and projects, such as the identity goals versus the goals of changing some other actions and projects. This work is particularly described in detail in the material on procedures and theorizing of dialectical-behavior therapy by Linehan (1993) and colleagues (Linehan et al., 1999). The working alliance attempts should be addressed at the systems of careers, projects, and actions, as well as in the interweaving of these systems that is interweaving of various careers, interweaving of a number of projects, and, finally, interweaving of various actions. Further, the relationship of actions to projects and of projects to careers must be clarified and worked upon.

Finally, all the levels of each of this system order (from steering to regulation) must be targeted and used in the process of building and maintaining a working alliance. For example, we know that by engaging in a supportive way in the patient's identity system as indicated previously, the therapist can achieve a better working alliance in dealing with other systems, such as the problematic relationship (Michel, Dey, Stadler, & Valach, 2004). Further, linking certain regulative interventions and dealing with action strategies with the appropriate goals helps in achieving informed consent, which is an important part of the working alliance. This describes in very general terms how the framework of the contextual action theory is applied to the issue of working alliance, which is further described in the following sections.

Linking Therapy and Life Processes

One way in which therapy and life process can be linked is by providing a space for an extensive client narrative. In the case of Mrs. Kirchberg, the therapist helped Mrs. Kirchberg tell her story by providing such a space, responding supportively, and recognizing and acknowledging the patient's identity goals and emotions.

Linking the therapeutic encounter, the therapy project, and the life project was also facilitated by Mrs. Kirchberg as she learned to address the issue of responsibility in the therapy project as well as in her other relational projects. She was treated as an active and important part of the sessions and the therapy project and not as a passive patient or victim. At the same time, she was able to determine that she played an active and important part in her own life, that she constructed her life, and that she was unique and best suited to live her life. She was given the freedom to decide on many issues within the sessions, learned to take this liberty, and to apply it equally in her life outside of therapy. The therapist's language changed from "what is worrying her" to "what is she working on now, what was she able to achieve, and what would she like to improve." Furthermore, the goal-directed organization of the therapy actions and projects became a link between the patient's life prior to and after the therapy.

For Mrs. Kirchberg, learning to act according to her own and joint goals during therapy served as strong link to her life outside of therapy. She learned to address her emotions in therapy and in her other projects. The tasks of connecting the goal-directed systems of actions, projects, and career prior to therapy, with the ongoing processes during therapy and with the activity which occurs after therapy, were facilitated by identifying the processes prior to the therapy as goal-directed actions, projects, and careers. Thus the patient was encouraged to build hypotheses on "goals she could have been following when engaging in these actions." Dealing with the patient's everyday issues in therapy and employing the processes the patient engages in in his or her everyday life provides the required continuity. The patient is not led into an abstract world using conceptualizations beyond the patient's everyday experience. Further, identifying those processes as occurring within joint goal-directed systems serves the same task. That is, the patient's issues are not used as indicators for certain mental or personality problems but as specific issues to deal with within the therapy. Additionally, identifying the joint goal-directed nature of these processes and their specific subprocesses, such as the steering, controlling, and regulating which applies prior the therapy, in the therapy, and after the therapy also strengthen the link between these three (see the following section). We exemplified this in discussing the issue of suicidality in which we outlined an approach to suicide as a goal-directed action (Michel & Valach, 2002; Valach, Young, & Michel, 2011). This approach mirrors therapeutic intervention as a goal directed process. This is a view which the patient adopts more and more thus changing from seeing herself as helpless to seeing herself as an active agent or actor in her life, that is, in her actions and projects.

Identifying Systems and Levels of Actions, Projects, and Careers

One challenge in therapy is for the therapist and patient to understand the full dimensions of the actions, projects, and careers in the patient's life. We address this as identifying systems and levels of actions, projects, and careers. Systems refer to actions, projects, and careers. Levels refer to the goals (the steering processes), functions (the control processes), and elements (the regulation processes) of the actions, projects, and careers.

Systems of Actions, Projects, and Careers. Mrs. Kirchberg's narrative indicates that she was engaged in a series of constructive, life-enhancing as well as life-destructive careers, projects, and actions. These included relationship careers (together with her husband, children, mother, father, sister, romantic acquaintance, superior at work, and others), identity careers (being female, sister, daughter, mother, employee, wife, housekeeper, politician, friend, sport woman, and so forth), joint careers (for example, as a part of the family of origin, siblings, family of procreation, and member of a political party), and careers connected to various issues (for example, achievement, sports, and cultural interests). She also engaged in destructive projects and careers (for example, taking responsibility for the family of origin, which she took on as a young child, to be a better wife than her mother and her sister, and the "failure career"). *"Because my thoughts were at home on how to keep the family peace, I did not concentrate at school, which made me miss being promoted. At the apprenticeship, my superior expected the best results from me at school, which I failed to deliver. He told me he was disappointed and then treated me as any other worker."* These careers—the constructive as well as the destructive—are also evident in midterm projects and short-term actions.

It is important to note that not all actions, particularly destructive ones, are consciously linked to the relevant projects and vice versa. Equally, not all projects are consciously linked to relevant careers. This was often expressed by the patient wondering why she behaved or felt in certain ways, in her lack of understanding about the connections between certain actions and projects, and even in her disbelief or resistance to accepting certain hypothesis about action-project connections.

Levels of Actions, Projects, and Careers. The identification of the specific levels within these systems, that is, the goals, functions, and elements of the actions, projects, and careers was exemplified in the issue of lack of energy

Mrs. Kirchberg mentioned. She complained about this lack of energy in the context of other depressive complaints and experiences. According to action theory, energy can be seen at the level of energizing actions, projects, and career. At the goal level, energy steers action. At the level of control, it is related to plans and strategies, and at the regulation level it is related to the unconscious processing of action elements. It is also closely connected with emotional processes.

In Mrs. Kirchberg's narrative, she indicated that the whole action, project, and career systems came to a halt because of lack of energy. *"I can't do anything (action), I am not interested in anything (projects), it does not make any sense, and I am indifferent to many aspects of life (careers)."* Thus, a number of threatening projects and careers were constructed, triggered, linked to, or actualized, paralyzed Mrs. Kirchberg in pursuing her usual actions, projects, and careers. The threatening projects and careers were destructive, detrimental, and emotionally undesirable. She was hesitant to invest her energy in them. In some way, the classic conflict assumption is valid here as well (we can paraphrase her situation: *I would like to engage in my work, but the emotional memory of a working project in which I was unsuccessful is activated. As I take this emotional memory for current action and situation monitoring, I am afraid to continue. So I withdraw my energy from this project, as the actions in the current work project become actions in the actualized previous unsuccessful work project. As I cannot skip this project, for some reason I just withdraw the energy*). As this happened in a number of projects and actions related to different projects, Mrs. Kirchberg felt blocked, caught, and in a cul de sac and subsequently disengaged at the energizing level.

Mrs. Kirchberg's resources for actions are limited because her basic cognitive (*I can't think, I can't learn, I am forgetful*), emotional (*I can't feel anything, I get panicky*), motor (*my arms are heavy, I can't get out of bed, I shake and tremble, I am clumsy*), and vegetative/autonomous (*I can't eat, my stomach revolts, I shiver inside, my heart pounds, I have diarrhea*) functions are limited.

She stated, *"All actions I can tackle lead to a state or in a direction in which I don't want to go, I am sure failing."* (We can paraphrase this as *"I cannot set up a goal as it would become a part of a destructive project. I cannot engage in a goal-directed action as I am following a destructive project which I know is not in my interest to pursue as it would damage other projects and careers."*) The energy issue was present at the highest level of the systemic organization of goal-directed processes, that is, at the level of goal and steering.

The issue of energy for Mrs. Kirchberg, although rational and accessible in her thoughts, needed to be tackled at a later time in therapy. It often involved helping her change the story, which she could not see differently as long as the identical, current emotions were at work. Nevertheless, the issue was addressed and it provided the frame in which the therapist and client were able to work, thus giving specific therapy actions a meaning—though it did not provide an instant cure. The therapist used paraphrasing, but initially addressed Mrs. Kirchberg's emotions and feelings. At this point in the therapy, the patient was more accessible, a change was possible, and the therapist and patient initiated change at the level of regulation, for example, through relaxation exercises.

Energizing Strategies and Plans. In this case, the therapist and patient did not initially talk about how the patient was to achieve her goals. Rather the therapist attended to Mrs. Kirchberg's emotions of dissatisfaction, frustration, and helplessness. Mrs. Kirchberg's words can be paraphrased as "*Whatever I do I'll be criticized, I will not earn the recognition from those whose support is important to me. I cannot do anything to achieve my goals.*" These unsolvable dilemmas, when addressed by social partners, can lead to disagreements if the goal is to solve the problem. Rather, the speaker, in this case the patient, wants the listener to attend to her emergent emotions and not to criticize, provide suggestions, or reproach her. Thus, Mrs. Kirchberg complained that people she spoke to told her not to worry and that she was mistaken in thinking that. However, all she wanted was to have her emotions and feelings recognized and taken seriously.

Regulation (the Lowest Level of Action Organization). Mrs. Kirchberg complained about tension, sleeplessness, and being flooded by strong emotions when confronted by a problem and when she responded impulsively. She was not able to provide differentiated energizing of action when it was necessary. In this and other cases, energizing follows pressure instead of being a balanced distribution or allocation following the goal-directed organization of an action. As a result, Mrs. Kirchberg was tense and her energizing was undifferentiated, comparable, for example, to the neurological constellation in the case of focal dystonia. Mrs. Kirchberg's energy allocation did not follow the differentiated requirement of action steps and elements sequence of the environment or personal requirement. For instance, her arousal level, increasing from the beginning of an action, was indiscriminate. It did not return to the basic level after several action steps, thus getting higher and higher and creating stress, anxiety, and tension. Such a condition limits the person's flexibility, rationality, and ability to be open to their problems. Thus, the regulation of action should be covered first in the psychotherapy as a major intervention, that is, following the usual intervention of providing space for significant narrative, supporting the patient's identity goals, identifying the patient's emotions, and developing a frame of understanding of the patient's problems. By making space for Mrs. Kirchberg's narrative, the therapist learned about her critical, destructive as well as constructive actions, projects, and careers, and he provided her with examples of the levels of the action organization following the problem of "lack of energy."

Intervention. Given Mrs. Kirchberg's complaints, the role the disordered energizing played, and the urgency to secure a proper functioning of vital processes such as sleep, as well as low accessibility of an effective intervention at higher levels of the action organization of the time of the first or second session, relaxation exercises were introduced. Following Mrs. Kirchberg's inquiry, progressive muscle relaxation (PMR) was suggested and a video of PMR was shown. Mrs. Kirchberg and the therapist engaged PMR (Jacobson, 1938) while watching an instructional video. After asking about the experience and whether Mrs. Kirchberg could imagine practicing this, the short-, mid-, and long-term benefits were described and a CD copy was given to her.

The short-, mid-, and long-term functions of relaxation exercises were explained in the following manner. The short-term benefits are relaxation prior to a challenging action or experience and relaxation after a challenging experience. The mid-term effects are creation of a space for being with oneself without pursuing external tasks and taking oneself seriously. Finally, the long-term benefit is lowering of the arousal level.

Mrs. Kirchberg's other vital functions were also attended to. After addressing sleep and relaxation, the strategy of learning how to stop rumination was given first priority. At this stage of the psychotherapy, a breathing and counting exercise was suggested and tried under supervision (during the first 90-minute session) and sleep practices were discussed. Later, the mindfulness issue was introduced, discussed, and exercised (Didonna, 2009).

Up to that point in the therapy with Mrs. Kirchberg, the therapist was able to provide a space for the telling of her narrative, to establish the connections of the actions and process within therapy with those of her life outside of it, and to identify the joint and individual goal-directed systems at play in her life. The next therapy task was to unpack destructive projects and careers. Emotional memory plays an important role in triggering the links to destructive projects and careers (see an extensive discussion of destructive actions and projects in reference to suicide in Valach, Michel, Young, & Dey, 2006a).

Addressing Emotion and Emotional Memory

The task of therapy is to restore or construct a life-enhancing order of emotional processes in actions, projects, and careers. Many psychotherapists strive to eliminate disturbing emotion without realizing their positive functions, as Greenberg and Paivio (2003) pointed out. Not all positive emotions are life-enhancing, for example, the good feeling engendered from alcohol or drug abuse can be part of life-detrimental projects or careers. Similarly, not all emotions that are experienced negatively are life detrimental, for example, anxiety or fear in a particular situation could be life-saving. Two interventions contribute to directing emotions toward life enhancement. The first is to insure that the patient develops a competency in emotional processing, that is, that he or she is able to differentiate his or her emotions. The second large task is to identify and work on negative emotional memories, which impact everyday situations and action monitoring. When a patient is reminded of a traumatizing situation experienced earlier, the emotion from the traumatizing experience occurs as the emotion of the action in the present.

A person's quick holistic monitoring of ongoing events, which has been attributed to emotional processes, can be deterred by emotional memory anchored in previous traumatizing experiences. Thus, an everyday situation in which others would feel only increased attention can become frightening for a traumatized person, with the consequence that he or she disengages from the ongoing processes in one situation, or copes anxiously in another, perhaps even in detrimental ways. Closely related to the issue of emotional memory impacting certain relevant actions in projects and careers is the problem of linking various careers in different areas of life. Contextual action theory allows us to see the connection between different areas of life such as work and personal life (American Psychological Association, n.d.). These connections represent the linking and intertwining of various careers and projects with different emotional textures, reflected in both the facilitative and successful engagements and destructive and unsuccessful ones. We assume and observe in our practical work and in everyday life that people are engaged in life-facilitating and life-detrimental processes. Although these processes are all goal-directed and, thus, follow the rules of top-down steering, the links between these processes can also occur as bottom-up steering often understood as impulsive or affective response (Valach, Michel, Young, & Dey, 2006b). Notwithstanding the importance of linking careers in various areas of life, it remains challenging for counselors to identify the relevant links and to help patients develop successful strategies when emotional memory is involved.

The following quotations from Mrs. Kirchberg are examples of the intrusion of emotional memory and the linking of various life-enhancing projects and careers to destructive projects and careers.

> *"This feeling occurred since my brother was brought into a hospital because of his alcohol problem and was put into a coma"* (trigger and a link to the family responsibility which generated the emotion of helplessness).

> *"I should have talked to him earlier"* (and help him to address his alcohol problem, which generated the emotion of guilt).

> *"My parents separated when I was 12 and I made it my task to hold the rest of the family* (mother and two older siblings) *together"* (career of family responsibility generated the feeling of being responsible for others).

Thus, in her family of origin and at an early age, Mrs. Kirchberg developed goals of being responsible for her family's staying together and for their peace. She then felt that she failed because her parents separated and then moved in together again. Her brother's hospitalization, an event in her sibling relationship career, was not only a sad experience of her sibling's health failure but also linked to her failure in her family responsibility career. It actualized feelings of helplessness and self-devaluation, among others. Mrs. Kirchberg's family responsibility career was threatened or challenged by the fact of her brother's health crisis and thus provided another experience of failure.

"After my parents divorced, my older sister divorced twice, and I was told in my thirties that my mother had an extramarital affair, I committed myself to a lifelong relationship" (setting up a "better wife" career). This career is threatened by the action of meeting the other man and their flirting project.

"I was criticized in my work" (trigger of or link to the failure career with emotion of failure).

"When my mother decided we should move back to my father's place I took it as my personal failure" (onset of a failure career).

"Because my thoughts were at home on how to keep the family peace, I did not concentrate at school, which made me miss my promotion" (failure career).

"At the apprenticeship my superior expected the best results from me at school, which I failed to deliver. He told me he was disappointed and treated me from then on as any other worker" (failure career). The success and working career is threatened by the failure career. Mrs. Kirchberg's failure career can be activated by taking on family responsibility, relationship, and work, among others.

In Mrs. Kirchberg's case, the failure career is activated in several relevant life areas. For example, she can be understood to have said, *"I wanted to concentrate on my own family (and forget about my brother); I wanted to be valued as an attractive woman; I wanted to be successful at work and develop initiative."* When the failure career is activated then the energy needed for life-enhancing projects was not generated and allocated. The activation of the failure career provided an emotion anchored in the emotional memory, and it replaced the adequate emotion of the here and now situation.

The patient described an important suboptimal strategy of employing or rather not employing emotions in her life, *"I put emotions aside and just functioned."* This is a complex issue that had to be addressed at all levels of the organization of goal-directed processes.

Intervention. The first intervention in addressing emotions was to help Mrs. Kirchberg identify her emotions and locate them in her everyday life. This included listing positive, neutral, and negative emotions and learning how to get from negative to positive emotions. Further, the therapy sessions included recognizing emotions in the therapy session; transforming anger toward herself to anger towards others; recognizing current emotions in everyday life; remembering positive emotional experiences; generating these experiences and the positive emotions; noticing emotion through mindfulness exercises and letting it pass if it was unpleasant; letting go of emotions without judging and thus avoiding unpleasant emotions; and learning the difference between action monitoring and anticipation of emotions in future problems.

By addressing Mrs. Kirchberg's emotions of shame in regard to her self-respect, she recalled her sister devaluating her political engagement. She also recalled the same feeling when her sister devaluated her skating performance. At the same time Mrs. Kirchberg recalled how her mother did not show any interest in her skating, which became very important to her, as it replaced her emotional life. Mrs. Kirchberg described her relationship to her mother as difficult. In the two-chair technique (Greenberg & Paivio, 2003), Mrs. Kirchberg was overwhelmed by her emotion while trying to talk to her imagined mother (in the third session). This emotion was reduced by a prolonged exposition in therapy by having Mrs. Kirchberg repeat her talk with her imagined mother several times (regulation processes) and then discuss the way this emotional memory impacted her current relationship and encounters with her mother. In the fourth, fifth, and sixth sessions, the traumatic experience of her father's suicide threat was dealt with using the technique described by Foa and colleagues (2007) for treating patients with a Posttraumatic Stress Disorder (PTSD) diagnosis. Mrs. Kirchberg was able to turn the self-directed aggression toward the environment and release it physically on a punching bag provided in therapy. In the seventh, eighth, and ninth sessions, she dealt with the traumatizing experience of separating from her husband when she was pregnant with their first child and her husband was engaged in another relationship, using the technique proposed by Foa.

Addressing Suboptimal and Detrimental Processes

In our view it is not simply a matter of trying to identify the systems and dynamics of the suboptimal and detrimental actions, projects, and careers as well as their links to the life-enhancing related actions, projects, and careers. Suboptimal and detrimental processes should be dealt with by jointly searching for optimal goals, strategies, and regulation processes in the ongoing relevant projects. In the case of this patient, this was about how to build up the encounters and relationships to mother, brother, other man, partner, and children; how to become a more independent and confident woman; and how to construct a new career or occupational security.

Intervention. First, after identifying the life-enhancing as well as life-detrimental projects and careers, Mrs. Kirchberg and the therapist determined how they were interwoven. In clarifying this, she was able to reset her goals in various actions and projects, for example, her relationship to her daughter. Specifically, she has two projects with her daughter: (1) that her daughter should have it easier than she did (Mrs. Kirchberg took over too many family responsibilities while too young and suffered a lot because of it) and (2) that her daughter should take on responsibilities.

Mrs. Kirchberg's daughter could read the first project well in their everyday encounters and felt that she was allowed let a few things go which got on Mrs. Kirchberg's nerves (the second goal is violated). On the other hand, her daughter internalized the rules of the project—it is important to take on responsibilities and achieve a lot—to such a degree that when she was not promoted in her sport team during adolescence, she developed depressive symptoms requiring professional treatment. In discussing her daughter's present situation, Mrs. Kirchberg realized that her daughter worked out a reasonable scenario and followed her vocational projects. This addressed the goal issue. Mrs. Kirchberg, realizing her conflicting goals, was able to relate them to each other in such a way that she did not continue to send ambivalent messages. Further, as she had a clear goal in mind when engaging with her daughter she was able to follow constructive strategies and refrain from a reproaching her daughter (plans and control processes). Her tone of voice was now peaceful and not full of her inner conflict (regulation processes).

In dealing with her relationship with her own mother Mrs. Kirchberg better understood the long-term development of their relationship, what happened, and how she experienced it in her childhood, later when she started her own family, and then when she felt under her mother's scrutiny and criticism. She was able to distinguish the emotion, she learned the necessity to let go of unfinished business in this relationship, and she learned how to effectively communicate with her mother. She changed her goals in this relationship, procedural strategies, and little details of their encounters.

Beyond these few examples, many of the patient's other constructive projects and careers should also be addressed. Equally, the issues of emotion, attention and mindfulness, energizing, steering, controlling and regulating, mentioned above, suggest how she organizes her actions in different contexts must be addressed. For example, learning how to implement attention and to secure the primacy of goal-directed processes over impulses are ways action organization can be addressed with this patient.

Conclusion

We addressed the five primary tasks of therapy from an action-theory perspective, provided examples, and now briefly summarize the intervention as it occurred in the 27 sessions. After dealing with the vital issues and regulation processes, the therapist and patient worked on some emotional memories and traumas from her encounters with her mother and father, identified and clarified the goals she developed in these encounters, and addressed how she was acting upon them in her later life and how she was going to change it. In the course of this work the patient developed a different view of her life projects and became more relaxed and interested in further developing her occupational career. This issue was particularly important to discuss, as the patient, like many Swiss women of her generation, did not follow the new social development of obtaining higher education. She worked successfully on her relationship projects with her mother, husband, and daughter. She worked on identifying and differentiating her emotional life and on becoming more mindful. This also taught her to become less judgmental and to become less sidetracked while pursuing her goals. Obviously, as the therapy was primarily conducted in the frame of the cognitive-behavioral approach, the dysfunctional cognitions were changed and several behavioral exercises were performed such as exposition (Otto, Smits, & Reese, 2004). However, for the purpose of stressing the contextual-action theory informed approach some other interventions are focused on. We would like to add that the application of the action theory in general and the contextual action theory approach in particular is not limited to the cognitive-behavioral psychotherapy. Comparable attempts have been described and are well known in psychoanalysis (Schafer, 1976) as well as in other schools of psychotherapy (Frankl, 2004).

The patient's transfer from the counseling actions and projects to actions in other projects was indicated not only in the patient's reporting feeling better, engaging in relationship actions, in following her own interests, looking after her inner life and expressing her emotions but also in experiencing the first setbacks when she expected more rapid progress; how she worked at home on her inclination to reproach herself; experienced success, positive feedbacks and feeling well; reported about her work on various projects; finding improvements in her relationships; building up more energy; and, finally, how she was able to deal with new negative life events such as losing her job. This might have helped her in looking forward and securing an interesting job, with a lot of opportunities for her occupational development about which she spoke in her final session. This issue is particularly important for Swiss women as it represents empowerment, allowing them to develop and pursue their own career, and not just taking up little jobs to supplement the husband's income. The patient's several years of experience in community politics during which she took up the office of the social department motivated her to pursue this area further and incorporate it into her occupational career.

As it is the purpose of this volume to illuminate the cultural issues in counseling and psychotherapy, we hope that after the cultural differences have been stressed the commonalities of the therapist and the patient will also be noticed.

References

American Psychological Association (n.d.). *Mark Savickas: Career counseling.* DVD. Series II—Specific treatments for specific populations. Hosted by J. Carlson. Washington: Author.

Constantino, M. J., Castonguay, L. G., & Schut, A. J. (2002). The working alliance: A flagship for the "scientist-practitioner" model in psychotherapy. In G. S. Tryon (Ed.), *Counseling based on process research: Applying what we know* (pp. 81–131). Boston: Allyn & Bacon.

Didonna, F. (Ed.). (2009). *Clinical handbook of mindfulness.* New York, NY: Springer Science + Business Media.

Federal Statistical Office, Neuchâtel. (2011a). *Divorce rates.* Retrieved from http://www.bfs.admin.ch/bfs/portal/en/index/themen/01/06/blank/key/06/03.html

Federal Statistical Office, Neuchâtel. (2011b). *Educational system.* Retrieved from http://www.bfs.admin.ch/bfs/portal/de/index/themen/15/02/data/blank/01.html

Foa, E., Hembree, E., & Olaslov Rothbaum, B. (2007). *Prolonged exposure therapy for PTSD: Emotional processing of traumatic experiences: Therapist guide.* Oxford, UK: Oxford University Press.

Frankl, E. V. (2004). *On the theory and therapy of mental disorders: An introduction to Logotherapy and Existential Analysis* (J. M. DuBois, Trans.). London, UK: Brunner-Routledge.

Grawe, K. (2004). *Psychological therapy.* Seattle, WA: Hogrefe.

Greenberg, L. S., & Paivio, S. C. (2003). *Working with emotions in psychotherapy.* New York, NY: The Guilford Press.

Gross, D. M. (2006). *Immigration to Switzerland—the case of the Former Republic of Yugoslavia.* (Policy Research Working Paper Series 3880).Washington, DC: The World Bank.

Jacobson, E. (1938). *Progressive relaxation.* Chicago, IL: University of Chicago Press.

Linehan, M. M. (1993). *Cognitive-behavioral treatment of borderline personality disorder.* New York: Guilford Press.

Linehan, M. M., Schmidt, H., Dimeff, L. A., Craft, J. C., Kanter, J., & Comtois, K. A. (1999). Dialectical behavior therapy for patients with borderline personality disorder and drug-dependence. *American Journal on Addiction, 8,* 279–292.

Martin, D. J., Garske, J. P., & Davis, M. K. (2000). Relation of the therapeutic alliance with outcome and other variables: A meta-analytic review. *Journal of Consulting and Clinical Psychology, 68,* 438–450.

Michel, K., Dey, P., Stadler, K., & Valach, L. (2004). Therapist sensitivity towards emotional life-career issues and the working alliance with suicide attempters. *Archives of Suicide Research, 8,* 203–213.

Michel, K., & Jobes, D. A. (Eds.). (2011). *Building a therapeutic alliance with the suicidal patient.* Washington DC: American Psychological Association.

Michel. K., & Valach, L. (2002). Suicide as goal-directed action. In K. van Heeringen (Ed.), *Understanding suicidal behaviour: The suicidal process approach to research and treatment* (pp. 230–254). Chichester, UK: Wiley & Sons.

Michel, K., & Valach, L. (2010). The narrative interview with the suicidal patient. In K. Michel & D. A. Jobes (Eds.), *Building a therapeutic alliance with the suicidal patient* (pp. 63–80). Washington, DC: American Psychological Association.

Müller-Jentsch, D. (2008). *Die neue Zuwanderung. Die Schweiz zwischen Brain-Gain und Überfremdungsangst (The new immigration. Switzerland between brain-gain and fear of over alienation).* Zurich: Avenir Suisse and Verlag Neue Zürcher Zeitung.

Otto, M. W., Smits, J. A. J., & Reese, H. E. (2004). Cognitive-behavioral therapy for treatment of anxiety disorders. *Journal of Clinical Psychiatry, 65* (suppl 5), 34–41.

Schafer, R. (1976). *A new language for psychoanalysis.* New Haven, CT: Yale University Press.

Schultz, J. H. (1937). *Das autogene Training (konzentrative Selbstentspannung). / Autogenous training; release of tension by concentration* (3rd ed.). Oxford, UK: Thieme.

Valach, L., Michel, K., Young, R. A., & Dey, P. (2006a). Suicide attempts as social goal-directed systems of joint careers, projects and actions. *Suicide and Life-Threatening Behavior, 36,* 651–660.

Valach, L., Michel, K., Young, R. A., & Dey, P. (2006b). Linking life and suicide related goal directed systems. *Journal of Mental Health Counseling, 28,* 353–372.

Valach, L., Young, R. A., & Lynam, M. J. (2002). *Action theory. A primer for applied research in the social sciences.* Westport, CT: Praeger.

Valach, L., Young, R. A., & Michel, K (2011). Understanding suicide as an action. In K. Michel & D. A. Jobes (Eds.), *Building a therapeutic alliance with the suicidal patient* (pp. 129–148). Washington, DC: American Psychological Association.

Young, R. A., Marshall, S. K., Valach, L., Domene, J., Graham, M. D., & Zaidman-Zait, A. (2011). *Transition to adulthood: Action, projects, and counseling.* New York, NY: Springer.

Young, R. A., Valach, L., & Collin, A. (1996). A contextual explanation of career. In D. Brown, & L. Brooks (Ed.), *Career choice and development* (3rd ed., pp. 477–512). San Francisco, CA: Jossey-Bass.

Young, R. A., Valach, L., & Collin, A. (2002). A contextualist explanation of career. In D. Brown & Associates, *Career choice and development* (4th ed., pp. 206–252). San Francisco, CA: Jossey-Bass.

2

Victim, Perpetrator, or BOTH?

A Child Soldier's Journey Into Healing Wounds of War in Sierra Leone

Ani Kalayjian

Georgiana Sofletea

Introduction of Authors

For more than two decades, Dr. Kalayjian has been on a journey of healing through forgiveness and meaning. Originally from Syria, an Armenian, Dr. Kalayjian resides in the New Jersey and practices in the New York area where she is a professor of psychology at Fordham University and president of both the Association for Trauma Outreach and Prevention (ATOP) and the Armenian American Society for Studies on Stress and Genocide. Dr. Kalayjian graduated from Teachers College, Columbia University, with master and doctor of education degrees. Additional specializations and certifications include board certification in traumatic stress, disaster management, trauma, eye movement desensitization and reprocessing, electromagnetic field balancing, and logotherapy. Dr. Kalayjian holds licenses as a registered nurse and as a mental health counselor in the states of New York and New Jersey with private psychotherapy practices in both states. Since 1990, Dr. Kalayjian has been involved at the United Nations (UN) where she works with several departments and committees focusing on human rights, refugees, women, and mental health. She is the author of *Disaster and Mass Trauma: Global Perspectives on Post Disaster Mental Health*

Management (1995) and the chief editor of *Forgiveness and Reconciliation: Psychological Pathways to Conflict Transformation and Peace Building* (2010), two volumes on *Mass Trauma and Emotional Healing around the World: Rituals and Practices for Resilience and Meaning-Making* (2010), one volume focusing on natural disasters and the other volume focusing on human-made disasters as well as over a hundred chapters and articles refereed and published in journals around the world. Dr. Kalayjian is extensively involved in several divisions of the American Psychological Association (APA) and holds many board member positions including chair of the Mentoring Committee and chair of the Disaster Prevention Committee Division 52, International Psychology. She has been involved in Division 1 for General Psychology, Division 56 for Trauma Psychology, and 48 Peace Psychology. She is currently appointed to the APA Task Force on Human Trafficking, International Division. It was Dr. Kalayjian's symposium on the *Taxonomy of Sexual Trafficking—Treating Survivors and Exploiters of Sexual Abuse* in one of the APA conventions that attracted counseling psychology student Georgiana Sofletea. After she found out that they both reside in the New York City area, a shared journey of collaboration in healing, counseling, international psychology, trauma, disaster management, and spirituality ensued.

Georgiana holds a bachelor degree in English with minors in biology and Romanian studies from Ohio State University and is currently pursuing a master of education degree in psychological counseling and a master of arts in mental health counseling at Teachers College, Columbia University. She is a clinical training coordinator and grants intern at ATOP Meaningfulworld. She possesses additional certifications or specialized training in progress: trauma and disaster psychology, American Red Cross disaster training, Gestalt therapy, and career counseling. Georgiana became interested in pursuing counseling psychology, and more specifically, multicultural and international counseling and trauma and disaster psychology, as a result of working with immigrants and refugees at the Community Refugee and Immigration Services in Columbus, Ohio, as well as from her own experience growing up in Communist Romania and as a refugee seeking asylum in the United States. Together with Dr. Kalayjian, Georgiana returned from a mission in Romania in October 2011 where they conducted an ATOP Mental Health Outreach Project (MHOP) on ancestral healing and forgiveness titled *From War to Peace: Transformation in Healing Generational Trauma* utilizing the biopsychosocial and eco-spiritual model (Kalayjian, 2002).

The case presented in this chapter is based on the data collected during a humanitarian rehabilitation journey sponsored by the ATOP Meaningfulworld (Kalayjian, 2010). Meaningfulworld has provided global disaster response through ATOP since 1989. It also provides training to paraprofessional counselors, disseminating outreach teams to over thirty sites around the world. Counselors undergo a series of trainings in the seven-step biopsychosocial and eco-spiritual model, a multiphase holistic and integrative healing method designed to ameliorate the effects of acute and chronic traumatic stress (for a detailed review, see Kalayjian, 2002). The organization is affiliated with the Department of Public Information of the United Nations and works closely with universities and other organizations to reach out to communities in distress and offer counseling, healing, resource building, and networking.

The Practitioner

Dr. Kalayjian is a pioneering therapist, educator, director, and author. She has devoted her life to healing those who have survived the devastation of disaster, whether human-made or natural. Her passion is studying the impact of trauma and helping others heal so that they can reach a state of wholeness. Dr. Kalayjian is frequently interviewed in the media for topics related to trauma. Dr. Kalayjian's parents were survivors of the 1915 Ottoman Turkish Genocide of the Armenians, Greeks, and Assyrians, which wiped out two thirds of the Armenian people (Kalayjian, Shahinian, Gergerian, & Saraydarian, 1996). Dr. Kalayjian grew up experiencing the effects of trauma through her parents' suffering, and that trauma became hers.

As a healer, Dr. Kalayjian has searched for ways and tools to best help surviving communities. Although she began her career in healing with a psychoanalytic model in 1989, shaped by postdoctoral courses at the William Alanson White Institute in New York, she later embraced the value of integration. As she began the mental health humanitarian outreach projects, she realized the limitations of the psychoanalytic school of thought. Dr. Kalayjian then founded two not-for-profit organizations, one addressing the humanitarian disaster outreach and the other addressing the pain of her ethnic Armenian community after the Ottoman Turkish Genocide.

When Dr. Kalayjian returned from her first MHOP in Armenia, she took a course with Frankl on logotherapy and expanded her theoretical foundation to include humanistic and existential psychology. She found Frankl, at the age of 96, to be extremely intelligent, humorous, and witty, and she was happy to have met him. This was a turning point in Dr. Kalayjian's life, and she tried to learn as much as she could (Kalayjian, 1995).

From 1988 to 2011 she organized and traveled to many countries and states to conduct MHOPs to help survivors heal: Armenia, Argentina, California, Cyprus, Former Yugoslavia, Kuwait, Dominican Republic, New Orleans, Texas, Mexico, Lebanon, Jordan, Israel, Syria, Palestine, Saudi Arabia, Sierra Leone, Kenya, Haiti, Niger, Florida, Japan, Korea, Taiwan, Sri Lanka, Pakistan, Turkey, Rwanda, and Congo. With teams of volunteer mental health professionals, she also trained professionals in those countries treating trauma cases after natural and human-made disasters and trained psychiatrists, psychologists, and general practitioners in posttrauma therapeutic interventions. With compassion, she has dared to confront the incomprehensible, providing hope that those who have been damaged can one day be made whole. More important, her ultimate vision is that through peaceful resolution, human injustice to other humans will be prevented altogether.

Dr. Kalayjian's effective abilities as a psychotherapist, educator, and healer are not only evident in her numerous international awards and recognitions but also from the client testimonies in missions and workshops around the world. Whether doing play therapy with children in Congo, holding a woman's empowerment group in Sri Lanka, healing boy soldiers in Sierra Leone, or seeing clients in her private practice in New York City, Dr. Kalayjian demonstrates warmth and empathy and practices multicultural international counseling in a nonjudgmental accepting way that inspires and heals those around the world.

The Case

Koroma, a 24-year-old man who worked a part-time job, spent all his days for a few years secluded in his one room away from his family until he connected with his aunt and began living with her. He was unable to face his relatives as all of his siblings and parents had been killed by the Militia. Koroma had been a child-soldier who was recruited by the Militia at the age of 12. The Militia told him that if he joined them, his family would be spared, but his family had been killed already, unbeknown to him. When Koroma was recruited by the Militia, he was attending a boarding school and, as a result, his schooling was interrupted. Based on Koroma's statements, it seemed that he had served in the Militia only for a total of few months; but it was over two years in this mode of serving in the Militia, escaping, getting caught, escaping again, and witnessing and participating in several atrocities. Later, with some other child soldiers, he escaped one last time and hid in a forest for a few years. Suspense, uncertainty, survival, and getting food and water every day were challenges he faced. He thought about running over the border into another country; however, he had heard that the Militia would even go across the border to capture escapees and subject them to severe torture and punishment, more forced drugs, and more suffering. Even after the war ended and the Militia withdrew, Koroma continued to stay in hiding for a while before he came back to his hometown searching for his relatives. He feared that the war had not ended and that the Militia was spreading the word that it had ended as a way to bring the escapees out from hiding. In addition, atrocities were still going on, which caused Koroma to be even more suspicious and convinced that he should stay in hiding. Later, a few of the children that were staying with his group came out and tested to see if the war really had ended. When they confirmed that this was the case, Koroma came to his hometown in search of his remaining family. The only family member he could find was his aunt. His aunt, too, was searching for her relatives. A third party told Koroma about this and reconnected them. Since then, Koroma has lived with his aunt.

Koroma heard from his aunt about some of the atrocities to which she herself was subjected. She told Koroma how his uncle had been killed. When they came to rape Koroma's aunt, the husband helplessly kneeled down and prayed out loud to Jesus. The Militia got upset, and after raping Koroma's aunt, they went to her husband and said, "So you like Jesus so much? We will then crucify you just like Jesus." They then proceeded to nail his hands and feet to a wooden makeshift cross, and after they nailed him, while the blood was gushing down, they set the cross on fire and burned him alive, while his wife lost consciousness and fainted. Koroma was especially traumatized by these eye witness accounts, feeling embarrassed and extremely remorseful.

Koroma heard about the ATOP team's arrival in Bo through a friend, and since many of his friends were planning to participate in the MHOP Training Program, they convinced him to participate as well. He appeared distressed, as his eyes were gazing to the ceiling, his forehead was wrinkled, his posture was slouched and uncertain, and his mood was definitely sad with some shame and embarrassment.

In this chapter, we refer to Koroma as the *client* because we believe that the term *patient* has too much inherent dependency, while the term *client* invites interdependence and partnership. Compared to patients, clients tend to have a higher degree of control on their healing journey and know which therapeutic modalities are a better fit and when they wish to terminate their healing process.

Koroma felt isolated from his community because many people knew that he was forcefully recruited into the Militia and had to comply with their orders for a few months until he was able to escape. Koroma hid for a few years and then decided to face his predicament. This decision was followed by the information about the MHOP. Therefore, when Koroma participated in the MHOP training, he was ready to address his demons, address his past, and overcome all his inner complications, as well as those with his community in Sierra Leone.

Although Koroma was only 24 years of age, he looked much older. Koroma's religious belief system was that of "born-again Christian." As he returned to the community, he was approached by a few pastors who convinced him that if he "found Jesus" and he was reborn, it would be easier to be freed from his past mistake of joining the Militia. This especially concerned the MHOP Team as war trauma and vulnerability were used to proselytize desperate survivors and force them to convert.

This method of taking advantage of vulnerable and traumatized populations has been observed in other countries such as in Sri Lanka after the devastating tsunami in 2004, in Armenia after the devastating earthquake of 1988, in the Democratic Republic of Congo after the civil war, and in many other countries. One of Koroma's concerns was lack of socialization, since he had to create a new family, as his family had been killed.

Koroma was physically healthy looking, although he was tortured by the Militia during the process of his forced recruitment. He was held in a small tank (the size of a coffin with holes for vents) for 2 days, with no food and water, and lying in his own excrements. This torture at age 12 traumatized Koroma and, as a result, his level of posttraumatic stress disorder (PTSD) was clinically high. He also complained of headaches and insomnia. He expressed symptoms typical to PTSD such as avoidance, hyper vigilance, nightmares, and flashbacks. The content of his nightmares were older men running after him with machetes and threatening to kill him, put him in a tank, maim him, or torture him. Some of his nightmares were very upsetting to him, as he would dream that the Militia were torturing his parents, that his parents were on the torture table, and that their muscles were being shaved off from their bones while they screamed in pain. This was what we heard from many survivors who witnessed the Militia torturing people and killing them slowly. Koroma, in tears, shared another method of killing he witnessed, which was cutting the pregnant bellies of young women while several members of the Militia, with compromised consciousness due to drugs and narcotics, made bets about whether their fetuses were girls or boys. Then they would cut open the pregnant women's bellies to see who won the bet. The fetuses were dead and they left the women to bleed to death.

The Context

The civil war in Sierra Leone began in 1991 and was not declared over until 2002 (for a detailed review of the events, see the historical report by the U.S. Department of State, 2010). Although war is typically a traumatic event, the conflict in Sierra Leone was particularly devastating for its civilians. Gross human rights violations occurred on both sides of the conflict, with the Revolutionary United Front (RUF) particularly noted for their brutal terroristic tactics. Adults and children were abducted and forced to join the RUF forces or face death (Maclure & Denov, 2006; Zack–Williams, 2006). Villages were frequently attacked, resulting in the destruction and burning of homes, schools, and health facilities. Civilians were raped and maimed, with body parts often severed. RUF forces engaged in cannibalism and ritual murder, with torture centers established throughout different regions of the country. By the end of the war, more than 10,000 people died and more than 2,000,000 were displaced (U.S. Department of State, 2010).

Children made up nearly half of Sierra Leone's population and faced the most severe consequences of the war not only as victims but also as forced perpetrators (Denov, 2010). Over 40,000 children under 18 years of age, the majority of which were boys, were actively engaged in the decade-long warfare of Sierra Leone (Maclure & Denov, 2006). While some joined as a last desperate act of survival, many boys were abducted by the RUF and coerced and threatened into becoming killers, combatants, commanders, spies, rapists, and servants. Refusal led to extreme forms of punishment, brutal physical assault, starvation, and death (Denov, 2010).

As the shock of warfare turned into everyday reality, young boys were told to sever the bond with their family and kin who were, more often than not, killed by the RUF and given no choice but to become dependent on the commanders who offered protection, promises of a better future, and, most importantly, a chance at survival. Terror, menace, military training, indoctrination, and cruelty guided acculturation into the social system of the RUF; brutality and killings were celebrated and displays of reluctance, fear, guilt, shame, and sadness were forbidden (Maclure & Denov, 2006). Young boys were turned into rapists, and rape was used as a weapon against girls and women and frequently involved multiple perpetrators, foreign objects such as sticks and guns penetrating in the vagina, and extraneous brutality. Sexual violence was often a daily occurrence and consisted of gang rape, individual rape, and object rape. Rape events frequently occurred in public, sometimes while the victims' friends and family were forced to watch. Young girls were also forced to "marry" young RUF boy rebels, serving as housewives or sexual slaves (McKay, 2005). The young boys received promotions and rewards for aggressiveness, and thus, successful atrocities led to a sense of pride, privilege, and belonging (Maclure & Denov, 2006).

The long overdue end to the decade of war in Sierra Leone led to the dissolution of the RUF and the livelihood and security of the young boy-soldiers crumbled once again. Thousands of children were permanently, socially, and psychologically traumatized, and demobilization and reintegration into society and societal norms was extensive and profound. The traumatic circular journey from victim to perpetrator to victim in the postwar context led many boy soldiers to feel lost, isolated, and fearful of recrimination and stigmatization (Maclure & Denov, 2006).

The Treatment

Before sharing the treatment Koroma received, it is important to explain to readers about the ATOP outreach team, the training they receive, and the preparation they conduct before they provide treatment. ATOP members are all volunteers and before they start their active roles in the organization, must go through a week-long, 6-day training. In this training, the volunteers learn about the seven-step treatment model, nature-made and human-made disasters, trauma, and how to run treatment groups to help individuals heal. In addition, before they go to a specific country to provide outreach, they participate in a 3-month long preparation work program. They familiarize themselves about the traumas in the specific setting, country conditions, socio-political-economic climate, issues during trauma recovery in the past, and the level of relations between nongovernmental organizations (NGO) and the government. They also explore possible governmental resistance the team might face in delivering the outreach (such as not approving the training programs scheduled by the universities) and decide what questionnaires to use to assess the participants' current psychological state and challenges. Finally, they establish email and phone contact with the local government, schools, camps, churches, and universities to inform them about ATOP and the upcoming treatment work that they will provide. Based on interest, the team decides where and how the treatment is provided. When the team arrives to provide the treatment, they usually stay from 2 to 3 weeks before returning to the United States. After the team's return, intense follow-up and individual work is provided both for ATOP team members as well as trainees from the specific country (through Skype and mobile devices) for a month-long period.

The outreach to Sierra Leone took place as a result of an American–Sierra Leonean NGO based in Texas contacting ATOP and encouraging the organization to go to Sierra Leone to address the trauma-healing needs individuals had and also the need for child-soldiers and people with handicaps to be integrated into their communities. The treatment provided in Sierra Leone was carried out by an ATOP team comprised of five volunteers who were born in Christian faith but practiced interfaith spirituality, and one Jewish volunteer. Although religious or faith alignment has been important in some other countries such as in Pakistan, Turkey, and Sri Lanka, in Sierra Leone the ATOP Team observed a special religious interfaith freedom, tolerance, and openness. Although there are many villages in Sierra Leone that have 80% Muslims residing, the larger cities are comprised of 80% Christians.

This treatment model was designed by Dr. Kalayjian in 1990, after the first ATOP MHOP to the then Soviet Republic of Armenia. At that time the model had only six steps; in 2008 the environment step was added on.

The seven-step biopsychosocial and eco-spiritual model (Kalayjian, 2002), through which various aspects of trauma, dispute, and conflicts are assessed, identified, explored, processed, worked through, released, and a new meaning achieved, incorporates various theories including psychodynamic, interpersonal (Sullivan, 1953), existential and humanistic (Frank, 1962), electromagnetic field balancing (Dubrow & Lapierre, 2002), learning theory, flower essences, essential oils, physical release, and mind-body-spirit chakra-balancing movements, prayers, and meditation. The seven steps are integrated throughout each healing session.

Step I. Assess Levels of Stress

Participants are given a written questionnaire, the Harvard Trauma Checklist, Heartland Forgiveness Scale, and other scales needed and used in previous calamities to determine the level of posttraumatic stress symptomatology and other trauma-related symptoms. These instruments have established validity and reliability, and they are short and effective instruments. Also added are questions pertaining to meaning and purpose in life, based on Viktor Frankl's logotherapeutic approach.

Step II. Encourage Expression of Feelings

One at a time, each member in the group (or in an individual session) is encouraged to express his or her feelings in the here and now, in relation to the disaster or trauma they have experienced. In postnatural as well as human-made disasters, the predominant feelings expressed universally were that of shock, fear, uncertainty of the future, flashbacks, avoidance behaviors, anger at the perpetrators or leaders, sleep disturbances, and nightmares. Among survivors of human-made disasters such as the war in Sierra Leone, those still traumatized experience predominantly the feelings of anger over the cause of the event and anger that it happened "to me" or "to us" and "not to some others," fear of recurrence, and mixed feelings over survival (happiness vs. guilt). The facilitator (a mental health professional), with a positive attitude, encourages the survivor to open the trauma membrane, dosing or titrating traumatic memory and its processing (Lindy, 1986).

Step III. Provide Empathy and Validation

Survivors' feelings are validated by the group facilitators using statements such as "I can understand . . . ," or that "it makes sense to me. . . ." and sharing information about how other survivors from around the world have coped. Also used is intentional therapeutic touch, such as holding a survivor's hand. Here it is reinforced that the survivor's feelings of grief, fear, anger, and also the joy of surviving are all natural responses to the disaster and need to be expressed. When trauma ruptures the individual's links with the group, an intolerable sense of isolation and helplessness may occur. Providing validation and empathy in such a group corrects these effects by reestablishing the mutual exchange between the individual and the group. Although survivors would prefer acknowledgment from their perpetrators, in therapeutic healing groups, it is found that validation, even though offered by the facilitator and not the perpetrator, has a tremendous healing effect, as reported by many participants.

Step IV. Encourage Discovery and Expression of Meaning

Survivors are asked, "What lessons, meaning or positive associations did you discover as a result of this disaster?" This question is based on Frankl's logotherapeutic principle: There can be a positive meaning discovered in the worst catastrophe (Frankl, 1962). It is also based on the Buddhist assertion that it takes darkness to appreciate and reconnect with light. Each member of the group is invited to focus on the strengths and meanings that naturally arise out of any disaster situation. Some of the positive lessons learned and shared in Sierra Leone were the importance of interpersonal relationships over material goods, the importance of releasing resentment, the importance of working through anger to achieve forgiveness, and the importance of taking charge of one's own life. The coming together of nations, communities, families, and individuals to assist restores some measure of trust or faith in self, others, and the potential for peace and solidarity. But this coming together is skewed—too many African nations or other developing countries are not represented, leaving out an opportunity to make sense of the extent of disaster that is felt again and again in these settings.

Step V. Provide Didactic Information

Practical tools and information are given on how to gradually desensitize utilizing the systematic desensitization process. The importance of preparation is reinforced and how to prepare is elaborated. Handouts are given to teachers and prospective group leaders on how to conduct disaster evacuation drills and create safe and accessible exits. Booklets are given to parents and teachers on how to respond to their children's nightmares, fears, and disruptive behaviors. Assessment tools are given to psychologists and psychiatrists, or in the case of Sierra Leone where there were no psychologists, to community leaders and professors of the university. Handouts and guidelines on forgiveness as a self-healing tool as well as for healing the conflict between communities in conflict are shared. Although forgiveness is promoted and addressed in all of the religious philosophies, ATOP's forgiveness focuses on the self-healing aspects of forgiveness as well as its positive impact in resolving intergroup and internation conflicts. This notion is based on Frankl's personal guidance to Kalayjian, who while taking a course with Frankl, was tormented by the anger and rage of the Armenian survivors of the Ottoman Turkish Genocide. Frankl asked Kalayjian to help the Armenian survivors forgive the Turks as a means of freeing themselves of the chains of anger and resentment and prevention of generational transmission of that pain and suffering (Kalayjian, 2010).

In Sierra Leonne, handouts were provided on grief, healing after a war, and how to take care of oneself as a caregiver. Also discussed were the restorations of rituals that were employed to deal with disasters in the host country in the past. Surprisingly not much was shared, and there were a lot of nervous giggles, indicating that all the indigenous rituals had been replaced by formal religions. They shared the value of coming together and singing, playing the drums, and community support. There were indigenous healers that one could visit, who chant, pray, connect with the ancestors, and share the messages of wisdom from the ancestors.

There is an emphasis in how spiritual practices and cultural rituals and traditions impact the process of recovering from trauma in various populations (Benson, 1996; Gordon, Staples, Blyta, & Bytyqi, 2004; Hedva, 2009), including Sierra Leone (Peddle, Stamm, Hudnall, & Stamm, 2006; Truth and Reconciliation Commission [TRC], 2004). There were no findings through the pre-assessment research about particular differences in spiritual practices, nor any information found on indigenous practices. But while in Sierra Leone, the ATOP Team was pleasantly surprised at how the different religions harmoniously coexisted and lived an integrated life. A Christian could marry a Muslim without mandatory conversions or without any big fuss. The team's host family, who was Methodist, had cousins who were Muslim and other cousins who were born-again Christian, marrying and living with one another without any obvious issues (more research is recommended to learn about this religious harmony). Additionally there were some indigenous practices for healing, such as placing a special rubber ring on the upper arm of a victim, such as Koroma, to ward off evil spirits. That did not mean that Koroma could not also practice his newly converted faith of born-again Christian. Therefore, a healthy integration of the traditional old methods was practiced alongside new religions in Sierra Leone.

Step VI. Provide Eco-Centered Processing

Practical tools are shared to connect with Mother Earth. Discussions and exercises are conducted around environmental connections. Ways to care for one's environment are shared, starting with one's environment and expanding to the larger globe, being mindful of the systems perspective and how we can impact our environment and how the environment in turn impacts us. When this step was utilized in Sierra Leone, we shared a list of mindful acts with the participants to help co-create an emerald-green world including ways to recycle, walking instead of driving, and being mindful of the clutter as well as garbage in front of Sierra Leonean hospitals, universities, homes, streets, and so on. The ATOP team began a beautification club, recruiting volunteers from the university. This committee remodeled the debilitated library of the University in Freetown, where the dust-filled books, old orange-colored newspapers, chipped paint, and bare windows were replaced by a newly painted beautiful room with new curtains and dust-free books nicely organized and displayed. Njala University Dean was very happy about the outcome of this project and congratulated ATOP team and the volunteer committee and organized an opening ceremony for the new library.

Step VII. Provide Breathing and Movement Exercises

Breathing is used as a natural medicine and a healing tool. Since no one can control nature, others, or what happens outside of one's self, survivors are assisted in controlling how they respond to the disaster. This is an experiential section of the model. Survivors are provided instructions about how to move forward and release fear, uncertainty, and resentments. In addition, participants are instructed on how to use breathing towards self-empowerment as well as to engender gratitude, compassion, faith, strength, and forgiveness in response to disasters.

In Sierra Leone, Bach remedies and essential oils were used to heal the body and mind. Dr. Kalayjian gave Koroma Bach Rescue Remedy—a flower essence used for working on the trauma, fear, loss, and helplessness of war. Bach Flower Remedies that are formulated specifically for trauma are made in England and distributed and donated by Nelson's Distribution Company. These flower remedies have been trusted for over 70 years in over 66 countries. Rescue Remedy, for example, helps alleviate the shock and helplessness of the trauma and contains the natural ingredients Helianthemum nummularum, Clematis vitalba, Impatiens glandulifera, Prunus cerasifera, and Ornithogalum umbellatum. Also given were citrus essences such as grapefruit, for engendering joy.

The group healing treatment Koroma participated in took place at a university in a large auditorium. People in the community were informed about the outreach. Koroma's friends encouraged him to attend the treatment. The treatment involved a two-day intensive workshop and follow-up individual sessions.

Koroma participated in the first day of training, where the ATOP team imparted information about the negative impact of wars, stages of healing from wars, types of healing modalities, integrating indigenous and cultural local practices, the knowledge from wise healers in the community, the spiritual belief system, their past experiences in coping and resilience, and so on. The morning of the first day included a lecture that was followed by a movie during lunch. This movie was a film created by ATOP showing different traumas that take place in different parts of the world emphasizing how people from all over the world cope with trauma. The afternoon sessions were the experiential ones, where the group members (approximately 70 each day) sat in a circle (divided into four smaller groups) facing one another and shared their feelings, while other members of the group expressed empathy and validation. According to Sullivan (1953), validation and empathy are the most important responses for recovery and closure after such traumatic atrocities.

As part of the first day treatment, the team also explored any indigenous ways of healing the group members may have been using. The group members responded with giggles and sarcastic smiles and indicated that they were brought up in organized religions and as a result did not practice indigenous ways of healing. However, they did share some methods that they heard from their parents. Some of these methods were speaking with an indigenous healer, chanting, or calling for their ancestors before a healing session took place. Because the group was not in favor of indigenous healing methods, they were not incorporated into the treatment ATOP members provided. There was only one cultural belief that some of the group members, including Koroma, practiced. They placed a black rubber ring on their arms and wore it for a year to ward off evil spirits and to prevent evil spirits from repossessing them. ATOP members respected this belief.

All too often there is no clear-cut point at which a psychotherapist can say definitively that in fact this is the healing point. There are many *aha* moments or insights that build one upon the other, to finally complete the puzzle perplexing and tormenting the victim. For Koroma it was his own experience of being forced into the RUF that had been tormenting him. On the first day of ATOP training, he learned about the negative impact of war and other human-made traumas, and he learned about ways he can practice forgiveness when people in his community ridicule him and tease him about his involvements with the Militia. Koroma, as a response to the community's reaction, was either secluding himself (such as envisioning himself going back to the torture tank of RUF) or being extremely aggressive and ending up in physical fights that resulted in extreme physical and emotional melt down. He was actually experiencing the typical response to trauma: Fight, freeze, or flight.

On the second day, Koroma came back to the training to learn more about how to forgive and the positive impact of forgiveness on the forgiver; he also learned ways to control his own emotions (EQ) as well as about the Spiritual Quotient (SQ). During lunch, another movie was shown, this one was *The Power of Forgiveness* (Juday & Schmidt, 2007), accompanied with designated time for reflection. During the afternoon group, Koroma shared an incident that happened to him the night before, after he left the MHOP training session. This is what Koroma shared with the group:

I was walking towards my house; well it's my aunt's house, she took pity on me and took me in. My coworker began teasing me and yelling after me "RUF, RUF, RUF," while pushing me around and hitting me. My usual response would have been yelling at him louder and hitting him back with greater force than his strikes. This time, I stopped, looked at him in the eyes and in a very soft voice, just like you taught us yesterday, I said to him, "I am sorry about what happened in the past; I wish I could undo it. I cannot change the past, but what I can tell you is how sorry I am, and I hope that you find a place in your heart where you can forgive me. I am already being tormented inside myself with guilt, embarrassment, and grief; I ask you please, forgive me."

Koroma burst into tears, while the rest of his group members were also crying quietly. ATOP team members were also in tears, but they began the empathic process. It was an emotionally moving session.

In addition to being a moving session, this also was a transformative one. Koroma continued sharing that the usual past dynamics of fist fighting led by anger, aggression, guilt, and embarrassment was now not only changed to empathy, compassion, and forgiveness but also that the two coworkers shifted so deeply that for the first time, they set down, talked, and called each other friends. When Koroma opened up his heart and expressed his feelings of guilt, embarrassment, and grief, it was the first time he had done that ever outwardly, and it really made his coworker listen and empathize with him, and then ultimately the coworker forgave Koroma.

As part of the treatment process, Dr. Kalayjian exposed Koroma to the ongoing process of healing. She often indicates to her clients that "healing is a continuum, a journey, which starts at birth and ends at death." After the two-day group treatment, Koroma had individual sessions with Dr. Kalayjian on the third day. Two individual sessions were carried out back to back, focusing on self-forgiveness as this was an area Koroma mostly needed to work on. He needed to forgive himself for the atrocities in which he engaged.

After the individual work, Dr. Kalayjian informed Koroma that she wanted to continue their work in the following month through phone sessions after her return to the United States She took his cellphone number and provided him with her landline phone number. For the next month, Koroma would call Dr. Kalayjian to set up a time to have a phone session and Dr. Kalayjian then would call him to carry out the session. Koroma felt validated stating, "I can't believe you know exactly what I am going through, no one else understands me." They had five phone sessions in which they focused on grief counseling (which is the fifth step of the seven-step healing model) and self-forgiveness. Koroma lost the most important part of his educational life when he was recruited into the Militia out of boarding school at the age of 12 and spent several years in hiding after he escaped from the Militia. He needed to do some remedial courses to finish high school. Dr. Kalayjian helped Koroma decide what he was going to do about his schooling and what steps he needed to take. They also discussed his career goals. Koroma decided to finish high school and go to college. The phone-session part of the treatment ended after a month. Dr. Kalayjian informed Koroma that he was welcome to contact her if something came up and also that she would like him to drop her an email letting her know that he is doing okay. Koroma frequently wrote to Dr. Kalayjian and informed her about his situation. The last they spoke, Koroma was attending college and close to graduating with his degree. Koroma thanked Dr. Kalayjian by stating that "at first, I did not want to participate in the healing program you organized, as I felt so embarrassed by my peers and the community members, but now I feel such a release, such a weight lifted from my chest and heart."

Evaluation of the Treatment

The atrocities Koroma shared shocked the ATOP team, especially Dr. Kalayjian, as these were exactly the same atrocities she heard of from her parents committed during the Ottoman Turkish Genocide from 1895 to 1915. Dr. Kalayjian thought to herself that almost one hundred years later, in another continent, humans continued with the same atrocities. What are we, humanity, doing wrong? Why is it that we are not learning the lessons? Why are we not mindful that these atrocities take several generations to heal and that they are unhealthy for us on the physical, energetic, social, and emotional levels? Why are we not mindful that these atrocities hurt us as well as our environment? While providing treatment, the ATOP members tried to deal with such questions as they came to their minds.

Crucial to recovery is the ability to find meaning in the traumatic event (Frankl, 1962; Kalayjian & Eugene, 2010a, b). MHOP trainings and healing groups helped Koroma find a positive meaning in his suffering; he said he realized that he had to go through this trauma to be able to strengthen his belief system, to be able to meet the ATOP team, and to learn how to forgive. Everyone in this world is exposed to trauma with varying degrees of intensity, some directly others vicariously. Certain personal characteristics and predispositions impact our attitudes of trauma and its continued negative impact: biological constitution, emotional quotient, social structure, past experiences of trauma, the culture, the geophysical environment, sociopolitical status, generational trauma, comorbidity, and so on. Unresolved trauma attracts and invites more trauma as a poor attempt to come to a resolution. Perpetrators, who create the trauma, in many cases, are those who have been traumatized at an early age by their loved ones, through abandonment, humiliation, rejection, and ridicule.

Forgiveness has also been identified as a way of coping with the effects of perpetrated, human-made trauma (Chapman, 2007; Kalayjian,

2010; Schaefer, Blazer, & Koenig, 2008; Staub, Pearlman, Gubin, & Hagengimana, 2005; Worthington, 2006), including in postconflict societies (Swart, Turner, Hewstone, & Voci, 2011) and in the Sierra Leonean population (Toussaint, Peddle, Cheadle, Sellu & Luskin, 2010). Although Koroma was able to somewhat forgive others as a result of the intense two-day trainings and healing group sessions, he confessed that he had difficulty forgiving himself. Forgiveness was defined by Dr. Kalayjian as the shifting from the automatic ego reaction (anger, self-protection, hurting back) to the nonreactive conscious response of empathy, considering that the other person is also a human being (Kalayjian, 2010). Studies demonstrated that forgiveness results in lower levels of posttraumatic stress and psychiatric morbidity (Friedberg, Adonis, von Bergen, & Suchday, 2005; Peddle, 2007; Stein et al., 2008). Failure to forgive one's perpetrators is shown to exacerbate psychological suffering (Worthington, 2006). Generally, forgiveness is shown to be higher in women and older individuals (Miller, Worthington, & McDaniel, 2008; Toussaint, Williams, Musick, & Everson, 2001). After a few individual sessions with Dr. Kalayjian, Koroma was able to reframe his trauma and forgive himself. Of course this is a process, and several phone sessions were made as a follow-up when the ATOP Team returned to the United States.

There were interesting dynamics, for being white Americans in Sierra Leone, as they called the ATOP members *poom wee,* meaning a white person. Although they said it had no derogatory meaning, rather that it had a positive meaning, as after we were called poom wee, the children extended their open palms wanting money, food, or a gift. Poom wees historically have been their dominators, or recently the NGOs coming from America or Europe always bearing gifts.

For Koroma, the ATOP members being white Americans (including one member who was Sierra Leonean–American) was a welcome release. They were not in Sierra Leone witnessing the war, they were not involved with RUF or with the larger community, so he saw them as nonbiased professionals from a distance, and since they were Americans (perceived as possessing superior education), his feelings of trust towards the ATOP members increased. In addition, since they were all volunteers, not only were they not being paid, but they each paid $4,000 dollars for the airfare and other expenses. This made a big difference to Koroma as well as others in the healing groups. Sierra Leoneans at large respected, loved, and put the ATOP team in a high regard for what they did, as they said, "You came all the way from America, traveling for almost three days, to come and help us? We are blessed!" Almost all survivors indicated that they were expressing their horrors for the first time to the ATOP team. Koroma said that he could open up with the ATOP team much more than he ever could in the past 10 years since the end of the war. He felt that the team would not judge him as his community has judged him.

Koroma's physical symptoms also disappeared, as on the second day of training he said, "This morning I felt I was the only one with all these nightmares and was hiding myself, but now I know these are natural feelings and normal symptoms, and that they will decrease as I embrace my traumatic past. I also came in with a lot of physical tension, headache, and shoulder ache, which has now disappeared."

References

Benson, H. (1996). *Timeless healing: The power and biology of belief.* New York, NY: Scribner.

Chapman, A. (2007). Truth commissions and intergroup forgiveness: The case of the South African Truth and Reconciliation Commission. *Peace and Conflict: Journal of Peace Psychology, 13,* 51–69.

Denov, M. (2010). Coping with the trauma of war: Former child soldiers in post-conflict Sierra Leone. *International Social Work, 53*(6), 791–806. doi: 10.1177/0020872809358400

Dubro, P. P., & Lapierre, D. P. (2002). *Elegant empowerment: Evolution of Consciousness.* New York, NY: Platinum.

Frankl, V. E. (1962). *Man's search for meaning: An introduction to logotherapy.* Boston, MA: Beacon Press.

Friedberg, J. P., Adonis, M. N., von Bergen, H. A., & Suchday, S. (2005). Short communication: September 11th related stress and trauma in New Yorkers. *Stress and Health: Journal of the International Society for the Investigation of Stress, 21,* 53–60. doi:10.1002/smi.1039

Gordon, J. S., Staples, J. K., Blyta, A., & Bytyqi, M. (2004). Treatment of post-traumatic stress disorder in postwar Kosovo high school students using mind-body skills groups: A pilot study. *Journal of Traumatic Stress, 17,* 143–147. doi:10.1023/B:JOTS.0000022620.13209.a0

Hedva, B. (2009). *Spiritually directed therapy protocol training manual.* Calgary, AB: Finkleman.

Juday, D., & Schmidt, A. (Producers), & Doblmeier, M. (Director). (2007). *The power of forgiveness* [Motion picture]. United States: South Carolina Educational Television (SCETV).

Kalayjian, A. (1995). *Disaster and mass trauma: Global perspectives on post-disaster mental health management.* Long Branch, NJ: Vista.

Kalayjian, A. (2002). Biopsychosocial and spiritual treatment of trauma. In R. Massey & S. Massey (Eds.), *Comprehensive handbook of psychotherapy* (pp. 615–637). New York, NY: John Wiley.

Kalayjian, A. (2010). Forgiveness in spite of denial, revisionism, and injustice. In A. S. Kalayjian & F. R. Paloutzian (Eds.), *Forgiveness and reconciliation: Psychological pathways to conflict transformation and peace building* (pp. 237–250). New York, NY: Springer.

Kalayjian, A. (2010). *Mental health outreach projects (MHOP).* Retrieved from http://meaningfulworld.com/index.php?option_com_content&task_view&id_179&Itemid_108

Kalayjian, A. (2010, August). Therapeutic modalities for victims of sexual trafficking: The biopsychosocial and eco-spiritual model. In A. Pipinelli (Chair), Taxonomy of Sexual Trafficking—Treating Survivors and Exploiters of Sexual Abuse. Symposium conducted at the American Psychological Association Convention, Washington, DC.

Kalayjian, A., & Eugene, D. (Eds.). (2010a). *Mass trauma and emotional healing around the world: Rituals and practices for resilience and meaning-making* (Vol. 1). Santa Barbara, CA: ABC-CLIO.

Kalayjian, A., & Eugene, D. (Eds.). (2010b). *Mass trauma and emotional healing around the world: Rituals and practices for resilience and meaning-making* (Vol. 2). Santa Barbara, CA: ABC-CLIO.

Kalayjian, A., Shahinian, S., Gergerian, E., & Saraydarian, L. (1996). Coping with Ottoman Turkish Genocide of Armenian Survivors. *Journal of Traumatic Stress, 9* (1), 87–97.

Lindy, J. D. (1986). *Vietnam: A casebook.* New York, NY: Brummer/Mazel.

Maclure, R., & Denov, M. (2006). "I didn't want to die so I joined them": Structuration and the process of becoming boy soldiers in Sierra Leone. *Terrorism and Political Violence, 18,* 119–135. doi:10.1080/09546550500384801

McKay, S. (2005). Girls as "weapons of terror" in Northern Uganda and Sierra Leonean rebel fighting forces. *Studies in Conflict & Terrorism, 28,* 385–397. doi:10.1080/10576100500180253

Miller, A. J., Worthington, E. L., Jr., & McDaniel, M. A. (2008). Gender and forgiveness: A meta-analytic review and research agenda. *Journal of Social and Clinical Psychology, 27,* 843–876. doi:10.1521/jscp.2008.27.8.843

Peddle, N. (2007). Reflections of a study on forgiveness in recovery from resiliency to the trauma of war. In W. Malcolm, N. DeCourville, & K. Belicki (Eds.), *Women's reflections on the complexities of forgiveness* (pp. 187–213). New York, NY: Taylor & Frances.

Peddle, N., Stamm, B. H., Hudnall, A. C., & Stamm, H. E., IV. (2006). Effective intercultural collaboration on psychosocial support programs. In G. Reyes & G. A. Jacobs (Eds.), *Handbook of international disaster psychology: Fundamentals and overview* (pp. 113–126). Westport, CT: Praeger/Greenwood.

Schaefer, F. C., Blazer, D. G., & Koenig, H. G. (2008). Religious and spiritual factors and the consequences of trauma: A review and model of the interrelationship. *International Journal of Psychiatry in Medicine, 38,* 507–524. doi:10.2190/PM.38.4.i

Staub, E., Pearlman, L. A., Gubin, A., & Hagengimana, A. (2005). Healing, reconciliation, forgiving, and the prevention of violence after genocide or mass killing: An intervention and its experimental evaluation in Rwanda. *Journal of Social and Clinical Psychology, 24,* 297–334. doi:10.1521/jscp.24.3.297.65617

Stein, D. J., Seedat, S., Kaminer, D., Moomal, H., Herman, A., Sonnega, J., & Williams, D. R. (2008). The impact of the Truth and Reconciliation Commission on psychological distress and forgiveness in South Africa. *Social Psychiatry and Psychiatric Epidemiology, 43,* 462–468. doi:10.1007/s00127–008–0350–0

Sullivan, H. S. (1953). *The interpersonal theory of psychiatry*. New York, NY: Norton.

Swart, H., Turner, R., Hewstone, M., & Voci, A. (2011). Achieving forgiveness and trust in post-conflict societies: The importance of self-disclosure and empathy. In S. Hermann, R. Turner, M. Hewstone, & A. Voci (Eds.), *In moving beyond prejudice reduction: Pathways to positive intergroup relations* (pp. 181–200). Washington, DC: American Psychological Association. doi:10.1037/12319–009

Toussaint, L. L., Peddle, N., Cheadle, A., Sellu, A., & Luskin, F. (2010). Striving for peace through forgiveness in Sierra Leone. In A. S. Kalayjian & D. Eugene (Eds.), *Mass trauma and emotional healing around the world: Rituals and practices for resilience and meaning-making* (Vol. 2, pp. 251–267). Santa Barbara, CA: ABC-CLIO.

Toussaint, L. L., Williams, D. R., Musick, M. A., & Everson, S. A. (2001). Forgiveness and health: Age differences in a U.S. probability sample. *Journal of Adult Development, 8*, 249–257. doi:10.1023/A:1011394629736

Truth and Reconciliation Commission (TRC). (2004). *Witness to truth: Report of the Sierra Leone Truth and Reconciliation Commission*. Avon, U.K.: Graphic Packaging.

U.S. Department of State. (2010). *Background note: Sierra Leone*. Retrieved from http://www.state.gov/r/pa/ei/bgn/5475.htm

Worthington, E. L. (2006). *Forgiveness and reconciliation*. New York, NY: Brunner-Routledge.

Zack-Williams, T. B. (2006). Child soldiers in Sierra Leone and the problems of demobilization, rehabilitation, and reintegration into society: Some lessons for social workers in war-torn societies. *Social Work Education, 25*, 119–128. doi:10.1080/02615470500487085

3

Counselling as Much More Than "Counselling"

A Case From Zimbabwe

Margaret Rukuni
Chalmer E. Thompson
Mmoja Ajabu

_____ **Introduction of the Authors**

Margaret Rukuni has a bachelor's degree in general studies (history and English majors, comparative religions and geography minors) from the University of Rhodesia (now the University of Zimbabwe [UZ]), another bachelor's degree in psychology (honors) from the UZ, and a master's degree in educational psychology (UZ). She is currently completing a bachelor's degree in gender studies (honors) at the University of South Africa. She earned her PhD in educational psychology from the UZ. She has also taken lifelong courses at the postgraduate level in psychometrics and research at Michigan State University and was a postdoctoral fellow at the University of Illinois at Urbana-Champaign.

Rukuni was a psychology intern under Mr. Latif, an educational psychologist and a counselling mentee at Lansing Community College in Lansing, Michigan. She worked for three years as an academic counselling specialist at the Zimbabwe Open University (ZOU); counselled for five years people living with HIV and AIDS with a nongovernmental organization called AIDS Counselling Trust and was its secretary and chair; and developed programs in counselling over seven years at ZOU. She organized and facilitated both the training of counsellors and counsellor trainers and developed training modules for the last 15 years. As part of these modules, she developed materials to be used in training rape crisis counsellors.

Her activism spans many years, focusing on women and children, and focusing on issues pertaining to HIV and AIDS, domestic violence and child abuse, and gender, as part of the Women's Coalition, an activist lobby organization for women. She belongs to the National Gender Forum, which lobbies the government to improve the lives of women and children in Zimbabwe. The issues they lobby for include making birth certificates mandatory for children as an aspect of their rights and advocating for the needs of single parents and their children. They also advocated for the passing of the Sexual Offences Act which was incorporated into the Domestic Violence Act. Rukuni is the current board chair for an activist nongovernmental organization (NGO), Women and Law in Zimbabwe, which is part of a regional organization. She counsels students on demand at the Women's University in Africa and is a member of the American Counselling Association.

Dr. Chalmer Thompson is an associate professor of counselling and counsellor education at Indiana University-Purdue University Indianapolis, United States. A contributor to the multicultural literature, her interests lie in applying scholarship to practice. Her foci have included racial identity development theory, psychotherapy process as therapists and clients address and make sense of race as an aspect of the therapy, and the integration of peace building in training mental health professionals in the United States and Uganda. Like Dr. Rukuni, she too considers advocacy an important part of her life. Thompson has advocated for legislation to prevent school dropout; regularly participates in letter-writing campaigns to end human and civil rights violations throughout the world; and, as a member of the Equity Institute for Race, Culture, and Transformative Action, provides Indianapolis teachers with training on ways to combat racism in the classroom. She cofounded the Heritage Project, an after-school and summer institute for school-age children that focused on culture and social justice, and is currently working with a curator and other activists (including Rev. Ajabu) to develop a summer and home-school project for children in Indianapolis, Indiana, which focuses on African heritage, math instruction, and critical literacy. She supervises graduate students in school counselling, and in the past, saw clients. However, much of her work with counselling and psychotherapy practice centered on process research, that is, examining the discourse of these interactions.

Thompson solicited nominations for therapists who practiced on the African continent and received the name of Dr. Margaret Rukuni of Zimbabwe from a close colleague, Dr. Helen Neville. Dr. Neville is professor of counselling psychology (and co-chair of this program), African American studies, and African studies at the University of Illinois at Urbana-Champaign (UIUC), USA.

Dr. Neville wrote glowingly of Dr. Rukuni, "I had the distinct pleasure of working with her when she was a Rockefeller postdoctoral fellow at UIUC from 2004 to 2005." Dr. Neville wrote further that Dr. Rukuni is responsible for transforming the field of counselling in Zimbabwe. "She developed extensive practice modules . . . [that] were helpful in training counselling students to provide culturally sensitive services to rural and urban community members. She also developed new conceptualizations of multicultural counselling competencies within the Zimbabwean context. While on her fellowship at the University of Illinois, Dr. Rukuni completed a project on assessing multicultural counselling competence in Zimbabwe and she developed a culturally relevant rape myths acceptance scale to be used in Zimbabwe. She is an accomplished scientist-practitioner, and it is not at all surprising that she has assumed leadership positions. She currently is the deputy director of the Gender and Research program at the Women's University in Africa."

Reverend Mmoja Ajabu was recruited by Dr. Thompson because of his 30-year involvement with the Zimbabwe African National Union-Patriotic Front (ZANU-PF) in the indigenous people's campaign to liberate the nation, then called Rhodesia, from colonial rule. Ajabu continues to work with the Zimbabwean government in its quest for economic independence. He was chairman of the International African Symposium of the Indiana Black Expo for many years. The Indiana Black Expo, founded in 1970, is now host to two of the major cultural events for Black people in the nation with international implications.

For these reasons, Chalmer Thompson, invited Rev. Ajabu to assist her in writing (with Dr. Rukuni) the Zimbabwean contextual portion of the chapter. Thompson met Rev. Ajabu when he was an associate pastor of Light of the World Christian Church and director of mentoring of Project IMPACT, a program for truant students and their families. They worked together on Project IMPACT and continue to work together on different projects in the city of Indianapolis. He is a graduate of the Interdenominational Theological Center located in Atlanta, Georgia, with a master's degree in divinity. Rev. Ajabu continues to be involved as an activist at local, national, and international levels.

The Practitioner

When resources are meager and the need for psychological care is compounded by a legal system that adds to the trauma of rape and incest victims, more is required of the mental health professional. The role of counsellor as traditionally conceived needs to be expanded (Atkinson, Thompson, & Grant, 1993). In this chapter, Dr. Margaret Rukuni shows how her role as counsellor *and* advocate is essential to the care of her clients.

The Case _____

Tracy (the family's names have been changed for this case study) came to my office looking very distraught and unable to clearly talk. She required some minutes before she could say anything. She had been referred to me for counselling by a former student of hers who knew Tracy as a member of the Seventh Day Adventist Church in Zimbabwe, a Christian denomination known to have structured systems for counselling.

In the case under description, Tracy's landlady's son is the perpetrator. The family of the children informed me that they had visited Family Support Trust (FST) for counselling but they did not want to reveal more information. Services provided by FST include pre- and post-rape counselling and provision of antiretroviral drugs administered by a medical doctor if the rape occurred within 72 hours. The parents informed me that the children in the case were not HIV positive at the time of their interaction.

The perpetrator in this case was around 18 years old at the time he allegedly started sexually abusing the first child (Rudo), who at the time was three years old, and he was a year older when he allegedly raped the second, younger child (Tsitsi) when she was two years old. By the time Tracy came to me with the case, Rudo was four years old and Tsitsi was two years and several months old. Tracy explained that she did not know that Rudo was being sexually abused for nearly two years after the abuse occurred. By that time, the children had been looked after by two nannies who knew that the rapes were happening but who had been threatened by the perpetrator's mother, the landlady of the cottage Tracy and her family rented. The perpetrator was an out-of-school adolescent, who under the laws of Zimbabwe at that time was both a youth and an adult accountable for his actions (Zimbabwe ratified the United Nations Convention on the Rights of Children in 1997, making the perpetrator liable to criminal justice for raping or abusing another child). Because the perpetrator lived with his parent, he was considered, even at age 21 years old, a child under customary practices. This may explain why his mother protected him using traditional practices that consider *children* as anyone who remains under parental authority, rather than defined by chronological age.

In terms of reporting, the two nannies of the children were more afraid of the perpetrator's mother than they were of her son, to the extent they refused to testify against the perpetrator when the case was before the courts. According to the nannies, the landlady threatened them violently, and in response, the two fled to their rural homes where, at the time (2006), it was almost impossible for the law enforcement agencies to bring them back to Harare.

Why Did Tracy Take So Long to Know Her Children Were Being Abused? As stated, Tracy and her husband Tatenda were lodgers of the mother of the perpetrator, living in a two-bedroom cottage on the premises.

The children's nannies lived with them in the cottage. The children had a fictive relationship with the landlady, calling her auntie, as is common in urban settings in Zimbabwe with regard to elders who are involved even informally in the care of children. The children were taught to believe the perpetrator was a *mukoma* or brother (or cousin) to them, therefore some-one to trust. Both parents also trusted him and did not imagine him to be capable of harming their young children.

According to Auret (1995), whether low, middle, or high income, the housing environment may influence the quality of care for children when their parents leave to go to work. For this case, being a lodger caused potential threats to the welfare of the two girls because both parents had to go to work, which left the girls in the care of others. Moreover, the cultural belief that children belong to the village may precipitate abuse conditions given the trust accorded adults (in this case, the landlady). Tracy had no clue her children were victims because the children did not tell her. Children among Shona, her linguistic group, are not taught to recognize when they are sexually abused. According to Chinyangarara et al. (1997), children can become victim to beliefs that are based on traditional practices (such as according trust and respect to adults); although, the authors admit there is no ethnographic evidence to substantiate this view. Tracy informed me that the landlady encouraged her son to rape the girls so that she could concoct some medicine (*muti*) to help her succeed in her business. Although I could not authenticate this allegation, Tracy believed that the landlady was advised that if her son had sex with a young child, she could use the semen to concoct medicine to obtain luck. The perpetrator confirmed this belief when he was asked why he raped Rudo. He did not show any remorse for his crime, perhaps because he did not take responsibility for his actions. His mother should have been implicated for abetting him, but Tracy believed she had bribed an authority who was powerful in the system. When asked why Tracy did not report her, she stated that she believed it was because the landlady used juju or some traditional protection against detection.

The Zimbabwe Traditional Healers' Association (ZINATHA), which represents some of the traditional healers, has a code of practice that does not allow any traditional healer to prescribe sex with a minor as a form of treatment (Chinyangarara et al., 1997). It is possible the faith/traditional healer who prescribed that the landlady ask her teenage son to rape the children was not a member of the ZINATHA because the organization has severe disciplinary measures against such conduct.

As indicated earlier, Tracy and her husband did not realize early that their children were being abused because the children and the nannies kept quiet about the abuse. The landlady had threatened them with harm and even death. The children were also bribed with food and attention. According to Tracy, who was eventually told about the rapes by her last nanny, each time the perpetrator raped one of the children, his accomplice (the mother, landlady) would cover the child with a blanket and perform some ritual on the girls. This included scraping the semen from the children's genitals to use as part of the *muti* and then bathing the girls, raising the suspicions of each of the nannies. When the nanny enquired why the landlady was bathing the children, she was threatened with death. The landlady, a mother too, was an indirect perpetrator who should have been prosecuted through the courts.

A further problem was that the younger child, though able to talk, may not have had the words to tell what had happened to her. In Zimbabwe, the Victim Friendly Unit (VFU) advised Tracy that it was difficult to press charges against the perpetrator on behalf of the younger child because of this issue of language. According to Tracy, when the second nanny tried to tell her the children were being raped, she did not believe her until she discovered that her daughter had contracted a venereal disease. As soon as Tracy realized her children had been sexually abused, she told her husband, who initially did not believe her. She sought the support of her church elders only to discover that not only was her children's innocence in danger but also her marriage. She did not immediately report the matter to the police. She confronted the perpetrator and his mother who reacted violently toward her.

Stigmatization and Bias One issue that arose from Rudo's plight was stigmatization that the child experienced at her nursery school. In one of our counselling sessions, Tracy informed me that Rudo was refusing to go to nursery school because her teachers were calling her unpleasant names because of their knowledge about the rape and warning the other children not to play with her. The teachers were making her feel she was to blame for the rape. I advised Tracy to talk to the teachers, and when she did, the name calling, according to Tracy, stopped soon thereafter. Rudo also was having problems playing with other children in the playground. When I asked her who her friends were at school, she mentioned that a cat was her friend. She did not understand why her nursery friends would not play with her any more. This made her very sad.

The other challenge Tracy suffered from was Rudo's maternal grandmother, who when informed about the rape, was quick to blame Tracy. She believed that the rape would not have occurred if Tracy had been home to look after her children. At one point, in desperation to be away from the school and community where the rapes took place, Tracy took the children to a rural home but discovered that Rudo did not adjust well there. Tracy told me that Rudo started wetting her bed, cried at night, and lost her appetite for foods she previously enjoyed eating. Tracy returned Rudo to her the cottage and decided to fight the stigma through the court. The younger child was completely ignored by the justice system on the mistaken premise that she was not empowered through language to give evidence. Tracy knew that there was an unfair bias against children who cannot verbalize their case. Likewise, it seemed to me as well that it was a travesty of justice that the case of Tsitsi, the younger daughter, was thrown out of court because of the assumption that the child could not explain what had happened to her. There also were signs to indicate that she too had been traumatized by her experience, such as displaying considerable distress when introduced to the anatomically appropriate toys and behaving precociously. The case also was thrown out because even though one of the nannies directly told Tracy that both girls had been raped, the nanny was not there to testify against the perpetrator. Both nannies mentioned that the ritual of washing the children after every rape episode happened to both girls, so Tracy had no reason to doubt Tsitsi was also a victim.

Another challenge that Tracy faced was her husband, who found it difficult to believe at first or even discuss the rape case with her. She requested that I have a session with the husband. First, I discussed with him the need for parents to trust their children and for both parents to be there for them. The goal of this session was to make him vent his feelings about the alleged rapes. He told me that his first reaction to the news was to look for a new home for his family. However, he had been reluctant to leave the place where his children were raped because the rentals were reasonable and he did not want any trouble from the landlady. That the children were in a dangerous environment that could result in repeated rape or secondary rape by living with the perpetrator had therefore escaped him. Mindful of the tradition of major family decision-making by males, although Tracy was very upset by the rapes, she waited for her husband to decide about moving from the cottage.

The Supports: The Girl Child Network and Other Relevant Agencies

Cases of individual children who are sexually abused are not publicized in order to protect the identities of the children. However, what is more typical is that the nameless stories of children are sensationalized in the media, so much so that the real life and ongoing trials of the children are publicly ignored or diminished. Thankfully, the Girl Child Network (GCN) rescues sexually abused children from family and religious environments that are toxic. As part of its advocacy, the GCN uses the media and any available forums to name and shame any person, group, family, or religious group that has sexually abused a child. The GCN's first director received a CNN award for her work. The rescued children are provided counselling, shelter, and education. The GCN has released information to the public about the horrendous sexual acts perpetrated on both boy and girl children.

Unfortunately, the providers of counselling services may not be trained adequately to manage very young children. One study in Zimbabwe found that only 6% of the 248 counsellors received any training. Of those that had, it was mostly in health-related situations rather than counselling in child sexual abuse. Often children face a lack of privacy, inadequate provider attention, and a narrow focus on reproductive health.

Childline is an organization in Zimbabwe that counsels children through a hotline telephone system. Childline representatives state that, of the 15,000 calls they get per month, 30% involve child sexual abuse, some of repeated rape, similar to the case described in this chapter. As noted by UNICEF, most children are sexually abused by people they know and trust. FST, mentioned earlier, is another nongovernmental organization that counsels and protects children from abuse. This organization has observed through its work that the perpetrators are usually stepfathers, uncles, grandfathers, teachers, or male domestic workers. FST sees at least eight cases a day involving child sexual abuse in the country, a frightening statistic where the HIV infection rate is one of the highest in the world.

Official police figures show that there were 3,448 child abuse cases in 2009. The VFC heard 1,222 cases of child sexual abuse, and it is widely recognized that a majority of these cases are not reported to authorities (UNICEF, 2011). Since 2008, there has been a campaign of zero tolerance for child abuse through the *Stand Up and Speak Out Information Campaign* run by the Ministry of Public Service, Labour, and Social Welfare; the Ministry of Women Affairs, Gender and Community Development; the Ministry of Education and Culture; the Ministry of Justice; UNICEF; and other partners, showing that there is some concern about child abuse in the country. About 30% of children in Zimbabwe are victims of sexual abuse. According to UNICEF (2011), 4,146 cases of sexual abuse against children were recorded in Harare, while three out of ten Zimbabwean children are sexually abused daily. In spite of the child-friendly judiciary system in Zimbabwe, Mutenga (2011) states that child sexual abuse is not only on the rise, but also that matters are worsening because of the lethal health problems and the threat of legal action; girl victims are infected with the HIV virus while others are killed by their perpetrators to conceal the crime.

In Zimbabwe, rape and domestic abuse are clear illustrations of some of the ways in which men exert control over women (Osirim, 2003). AfricanFathers in Zimbabwe, an NGO, admits that the role of fathers in providing social protection to children has largely been missing, accounting for some of the sexual violence against children.

International Conventions on the Child

Child abuse should not be tolerated. Children have rights as determined under the Convention on the Rights of the Child (CRC) (November 1989) that describes the rights entitlement of every child including nondiscrimination on the basis of sex, provides for protection from all forms of sexual exploitation and abuse, obliges states to protect children from sexual exploitation and abuse, and obliges states to take measures to reintegrate children who have suffered Sexual Gender Based Violence (SGBV) into society. SGBV includes rape and incest, which seem to be at alarming levels in Zimbabwe. Zimbabwe is a signatory to the CRC as well as to the

African Charter on the Rights and Welfare of the Child (ACRWC, 1995) that defines the age of a child as 18 years and under; entitles children to protection from exploitation, abuse, trafficking, abduction, and sexual exploitation; and binds states to action once they ratify the charter. These two instruments obligate Zimbabwe to protect all children. Government ministries that are empowered to protect children are the Ministry of Health and Child Welfare and the Ministry of Labour and Social Welfare, although the Ministry of Education, Arts, Sports, and Culture is responsible for child welfare for most children from the age of 3 years old.

The Context

The following information was derived from the U.S. Department of State Fact Sheet on Zimbabwe (2011) unless otherwise noted. The Republic of Zimbabwe is a landlocked country in southern Africa, bordered by the Zambezi and Limpopo rivers. The official language is English. However, the majority of the population speaks Shona, spoken by the Mashona people who constitute 75% of the population, while the second vernacular language spoken is Ndebele of the Matabele people who constitute about 20% of the population. Afrikaners from South Africa, the Portuguese from Mozambique, and White immigrants from England, make up the remaining population. Zimbabwe has one of the highest literacy rates in Africa at 91%. There are about 11 million people living in the country. Although Zimbabwe offers popular tourist attractions in Victoria Falls, Great Zimbabwe, and selected game parks, much of the country's infrastructure remains depressed and emergency medical care is limited.

In 1980, Zimbabwe won its independence from Britain after a liberation war. One of the major issues for the liberation war was land largely owned by descendants of White settlers. Under the Lancaster House Agreement, the document that denoted the liberation of Zimbabwe from Britain, the Zimbabwean Government distributed some of the land from White farmers to landless Black farmers on a willing buyer selling basis. The Lancaster House Constitution expired in 1990, following which the Government of Zimbabwe amended the constitution in order to accommodate compulsory acquisition of land from White farmers. In 2000, the government of Zimbabwe commenced a fast-track land program that attracted sanctions from the Western countries such as the United States. In 2008, following a hotly contested election, the three major political parties signed the Global Political Agreement, which led to the formation of a Government of National Unity in February, 2009. The inclusive government had hoped for the removal of the sanctions, but instead, the Western Governments have renewed the sanctions annually while providing humanitarian assistance to the ordinary Zimbabwean. The influence of the sanctions on Zimbabwean development and infrastructure has been devastating (Moyo, 2011; United Nations Security Council, 2008). Services deteriorated, for example, water and electricity were in short supply, and cholera broke out in many urban centers. Many families could not easily access health services (United Nations Human Development Report, 2010).

Counselling in Context

As a counsellor trainer at a local university, I, Dr. Rukuni, always wondered how counselling was perceived by Zimbabweans as well as how it was practiced, considering that students of counselling programmes learned counselling techniques developed in Euro-American contexts. Therefore, they practiced principles and techniques borrowed from contexts quite unlike Zimbabwe and at most were required to adopt a multicultural perspective. To find out how Zimbabweans perceived the counselling profession, I requested a prominent television talk show presenter to hold a discussion on the issue in 2006 with the Zimbabwean television public. A group of both urban and rural men and women was invited to the Zimbabwe Broadcasting Television to discuss whether they would consult a professional counsellor to provide counselling services to any of them. Among the audience of twenty people were three traditional healers, two Christian pastors, and five women who were regular supporters of the talk show. One health concern that popularized the word *counselling* in Zimbabwe is the HIV and AIDS pandemic that is still ravaging the country. One reason that has been blamed for children being vulnerable to sexual abuse is the desperate economic situation, the worst period being from 2006 to 2010, including the period when the case of Tracy (described in the previous section) falls. In addition, high inflation forced many women to look for work and leave their children unattended at home. There are many training workshops on aspects of counselling ranging from 2-day sessions to degree programmes run at institutions of higher learning. To the lay person, the word *counselling* is associated with HIV and AIDS and most training previously provided was on home-based care. The television audience stated overwhelmingly that they would not seek services from professional counsellors since they are strangers. They preferred to use family members who would use Shona or Ndebele (the main languages spoken by more than 96% of Zimbabwe). One participant stated that publicising one's illness to a stranger is like "lifting your armpits and letting others smell them" which figuratively means exposing oneself, because many in Zimbabwe believe it is not necessary to reveal family secrets to strangers. Illness among the Shona is a close family affair that should not be discussed in public, and a counsellor, being a stranger, should not be privy to a family's private affairs. The audience considered Western-trained counsellors to hold foreign ideas and methods and more likely to ignore their beliefs and systems.

Apart from the college- and university-trained counsellors in Zimbabwe, many counsellors were trained within a medical model that focused on HIV and AIDS. Until 2002, one counsellor training school popular in Zimbabwe was a centre (training and counselling) linked to the UK Tavistock School called the CONNECT Institute, which uses psychodynamic techniques. Although it also provides counselling services to children and families, it caters mainly to elite (i.e., wealthy) groups. The effectiveness of traditional methods of counselling has not been adequately researched by indigenous researchers, nor the multicultural issues that affect counselling been explored in depth.

The Treatment

The counselling proffered to Tracy, her husband, and the two girls involved contact with each family member individually. It also entailed couples counselling as well as regular contact with the Victim Friendly Courts (VFC), described in detail in the following section.

Victim Friendly Courts

As mentioned earlier, by the time Tracy approached me for help through counselling, she had been counselled by the FST and she had her girls counselled by the Victim Friendly Unit (VFU). The latter has men and women trained in counselling, mainly in systemic counselling techniques. The VFU is expected to assist victims of sexual abuse through humane and sensitive interviewing. One observation made by members of the GCN based on their experiences with the VFU is that the counselling skills that should protect the victims of sexual abuse are sometimes less than desired. Sometimes the child is subjected to secondary rape through repeated appearances before the courts or delays in handling the case. There also is the possibility of the child refusing to cooperate either because the child wants to forget an incident or rape incidents that have traumatised him or her.

The VFU investigators are supposed to be sensitive, friendly, and empathetic. For the very young child, such as Rudo, confronting the perpetrator is out of the question. The VFU is trained to use technology, such as the video camera, for the child to identify the perpetrator in a safe room. Sometimes these useful gadgets do not work. My experience was that for the six times we waited in this room with Tracy and her children in 2006, none of the videos worked. The toys in the room were too old, and the use of anatomically accurate dolls seemed to retraumatise the children. Rudo would not play, touch, or even look at the dolls. We instead had to bring books of animals or chant Shona songs about the animals on the murals on the walls in one of the waiting rooms. We waited for hours before any of the VFU staff would attend to us.

In my presence, the VFU personnel asked the child to explain in detail what the *mukoma* (brother) or the perpetrator did to her. I observed that not one of the men and women was sensitive to the fact that he or she was inflicting secondary rape on the child. The mother complained several times to the senior prosecutor that the VFU members were upsetting the child. Each day the child was left with her mother and sometimes with me for hours, with the few bursts of activity when she was asked the same questions. The mother informed me after such sessions that the child would be restless at night, wet her bed, or refuse to go to nursery school the following day. Although it is difficult to establish a causal link between the court sessions and bed wetting, it is possible that meting out justice as quickly as possible would have been justice served. Strictly, the victim should have been aided by the state as soon as the case was reported to the police.

The VFC is a noble idea that has its challenges, but at the time of this case, there was more frustration than relief to the child and her family. Although the VFU is expected to provide transport to victims, the family had to pay for the medical expenses and transport expenses each time they were called to attend the court sessions. The longer the case dragged on, the more costs the family incurred psychologically, emotionally, and financially. According to UNICEF (2011), the Zero Tolerance against Child Abuse campaign started in 2003 could go a long way to fight child abuse if the VFC were present in all the provinces. Unfortunately, the VFU is spread too thin in Zimbabwe and may not have enough resources to train its personnel. One complaint from the Women's Coalition, a combination of women's organisations and individuals, is that there is not a lot of progress in training police in the use of counselling or at the very least, in supplying them with knowledge to help better assist rape and sexual violence victims.

Individual and Couple Sessions

When I had a session with Tatenda and Tracy together, there were other marital issues that interfered with focusing on the rape case. Eventually, they agreed that it was important to focus on the rape case together and bracket any negative feelings they had for each other. Tatenda promised that they would use their church elders for what he believed were marital issues, separate from parental concerns for their children. Once that matter was settled, my plan was to help the couple act promptly to protect and support their children.

The third individual session with Tracy seemed less tense and I enquired about the change in outlook. Tracy was happy because her husband had decided to give her all the necessary support for moving on in their lives. For example, Tatenda agreed that they would move out of the low-density (in population) suburb to a high-density suburb where it would be easier to find a nanny to look after the children. More importantly, they moved the children to a different nursery school where the children were not ostracised for their experience. They later returned to Harare.

Sessions With Rudo, the Older Child

There were three sessions that I concentrated on with Rudo in order to help her regain self-esteem from the rapes and the secondary traumas surrounding the legal process. As earlier noted, I allowed Rudo to read English and Shona books that had animal stories as a way to prompt disclosure from the child. Sometimes I played games that Rudo liked that were in her language, such as playing out the story of the clever hare and foolish baboon. The pictures were helpful. The mother reported how Rudo would later retell the stories to her younger sister. The parents did not use English language as their normal language of communication with their children or each other, so the English stories were new and not easy to understand. Helping Rudo be more playful and engaging in her own language proved helpful in restoring her self-esteem.

Helping children make sense out of violent behaviour is difficult and Rudo needed the opportunity to ask questions about her victimization, initially by her perpetrator and later by other adults as well as nursery school children. Rudo wanted to know why she had to explain to the prosecutor or the VFU persons what had happened to her. Slowly I explained to her that the person who had raped her had to be brought before justice, and that he was the one who was wrong, not her or her sister. I wanted her to know she was innocent and the perpetrator was the one who had wronged her. When she detailed how the other children were laughing at her for the rape, she needed to hear that these people had no right to treat her that way.

Rudo also wanted to know what would happen to her if the perpetrator was to see her. Would he harm her? She feared being raped again. I observed that she had to relearn to trust people, including her father and mother. She was unusually worried for her sister, something we also discussed. She needed reassurance that she was like every child and must be allowed to be a child. We went over several times each session why it was important for her to continue to answer the questions from the VFU. Rudo would repeat that mukoma was a bad person who should not be allowed to hurt any other children. She described in detail how exactly the perpetrator raped her, calling his penis *chinhu chake* (translated, his thing). In my time with her, I made no attempt to identify the rapist's genitalia using explicit language in Shona. The Shona do not discuss sex with children as young as Rudo. It is taboo. It also is important to note that the use of anatomically accurate dolls poses a predicament because of the taboo of eliciting any discussion related to sex with children at this young age.

Reflexivity

The first three sessions with the child (Rudo) left me exhausted and with misgivings about the treatment. For example, I worried that I was also intruding into the family's life, especially when giving some attention to the parents' issues. I felt that perhaps concentrating on the child was what I should do, but realized I needed both parents to be supportive of each other and the children. I believed the children should not see or hear their parents arguing or quarrelling, otherwise they would think they were to blame. Instead of spending 50 minutes per session, I had longer sessions with the children.

Once I knew the child was able to testify on camera, I sometimes felt that the process was too protracted because the system ignored the likelihood that each court session could retraumatise Rudo. I wrote a letter to the senior prosecutor to protest against this insensitivity to the child and her family, which may explain the increased pace in setting up court sessions. Even that was not fast enough. Twice Tracy, Tatenda, and I tried to meet with the senior prosecutor but had little success. Finally, Tracy told me that after her request that the case find closure, the perpetrator was sentenced to 12 months in a penitentiary. As noted earlier, the mother was not prosecuted. These outcomes were not satisfactory, especially since the case had taken so long to be tried. Due process did not seem to have taken place. In spite of this poor showing of justice, that the perpetrator was tried and sentenced was something. When I asked how she felt about the sentence, Tracy responded that at least the perpetrator was in jail. That factor alone to her was good enough.

Evaluation of the Treatment

What was the nature of my counselling relationship with the child and her parents? The eclectic counselling approach was adopted because it did not demand conformity to some theory but rather allowed me to concern myself with the varied needs of Rudo and her parents. For example, it was important to develop a friendly approachable relationship, especially with the child and the parents. I needed the parents to trust that whatever I did with the child was safe, that I behaved ethically, and that I did not do any more harm to the child. I strove to gain the child's trust before asking her to describe what had happened to her. I could not replace the child's parents, but I had to be seen by the child as protecting her from possible harm. I debriefed with another counsellor when transference and countertransference issues intervened in the counselling relationship. As an anti-rape activist, I had to strike a balance so that this role did not intrude into my thoughts when in the counselling relationship with the child. I was often conscious of the language I used with the child and her parents. Whenever the VFU personnel spoke to the child when I was present, I did not participate. I believe my presence in the room modified how they interacted with the child.

In hindsight, I did not quite adopt any specific counselling theories, such as behaviourism or psychoanalysis as I learned them or taught others. There was however, respect for the humanity (*hunhu or ubuntu*) toward the clients, and the goal that I achieve the best outcomes for them was important. I tried to integrate my values and beliefs with those of my clients. I agree with Norcross, Hedges, and Prochaska, (2002) who stated that the major challenge for the field of psychotherapy will be "to discover creative ways to integrate the values and worldviews of multiple cultures within the discourse of efficiency and evidence that currently dominate health care" (cited in Corey, 2011, p. 274). What seemed to work was adopting a technical eclectic approach, allowing for use of some key principles and concepts from different theories. For example, Tracy was able to address the patriarchal problems of her husband, who tended to blame her as a failing mother. In Shona culture, this confrontation is a serious violation of women's relationship to men, especially from one who is believed to be a responsible mother and Christian. From a feminist counselling position, Tracy and I were able to clarify some of the underlying sources of her husband's reluctance to accept that the perpetrator was to blame for violating his daughters and that both parents had to trust the daughters. This clarification helped prompt needed action by Tracy.

I strove to be congruent, empathetic, and to provide unconditional positive regard to the children in order to build trust and raise the children's self-esteem, concepts drawn from Carl Rogers's person-centered counselling approach. These facilitative conditions were important in my work with Tracy, for she had to be assisted to believe she was not to blame for the rapes. Because of the extent of problems pertaining to the rapes, most prominently the societal crisis surrounding the abuse of (especially) girl children, it honestly was challenging to identify concepts from the theories I have learned about in my life-long education as a practitioner and activist. Tracy had to deal with the realities of her patriarchal culture. Because we worked through those issues over several sessions together, my satisfaction with the outcome of the case was that we had a relationship that allowed healing to take place, rather than resort to some distinct theoretical stance. From an existential standpoint, I believed I was there for the family because they could call me and talk on the telephone or face-to-face whenever they needed. We developed a trusting relationship that allowed effective therapeutic counselling to take place. Sometimes it was necessary to take a directive approach, other times the client took charge of the healing process.

Conclusion

The experiences chronicled in this chapter are based on an actual series of events centered on the repeated rape of two children who were traumatized. Because of space limitations, I concentrated my attention on the oldest child, Rudo, as well as her parents. It is true that some child rape cases never get reported, or if they do, are never tried to completion (where the perpetrator is arrested, tried, and convicted). From this counselling experience, I have learned never to take for granted how wise and resilient children can be. The justice system is not that simple. I wondered why the boy raped two children, worse still, why the mother of the perpetrator was insensitive to the trauma inflicted on the young children. As Corey (2011) states, it is important to have a systematic, consistent, personal, and disciplined approach to counselling that integrates the cultural values of both the counsellor and counselled. The expression, "the context defines how you counsel," makes this counselling experience both therapeutic and unique. Both the counsellor and the counselled experienced the rape of the child in different ways that both victimized them and made them survivors.

Rudo is now in grade five at a primary school; hopefully she has survived her ordeal.

References

Atkinson, D. R., Thompson, C. E., & Grant, S. K. (1993). A three-dimensional model for counselling racial/ethnic minorities. *The Counselling Psychologist, 21,* 257–277.

Auret, D. (1995). *Urban housing: A national crisis? Overcrowded and inadequate housing and the social and economic effects.* Gweru, Zimbabwe: Mambo.

Chinyangara, I., Chokuwenga, I., Dete, R., Dube, L., Kembo, J., Moyo, P., & Nkomo, R. (1997). Indicators for children's rights: Zimbabwe country case study. Retrieved from http://childabuse.com/childhouse/childwatch/cwi/projects/indicators/Zimbabwe/ind_zim_ch4.html

Corey, G. (2011). Designing an integrative approach to counselling practice. *Article 29 ACA Vistas ACA Online Library,* http://www.counselling.org/

Moyo, T. (2011, October 18). We need other power sources. *The Herald.* Retrieved from http://www.herald.co.zw/index.php?option=com_content&view=article&id=24023%3Awe-need-other-power-sources&Itemid=129

Mutenga, T. (2011, August 3). Zimbabwe: Child sexual abuse on the rise. *The Financial Gazette.* Retrieved from http://allafrica.com/stories/201108081194.html

Norcross, J. C., Hedges, M., Prochaska, J. O. (2002). The face of 2010: A Delphi poll on the future of psychotherapy. *Professional Psychology: Research and Practice, 33,* 316–322.

Osirim, M. J. (2003). Crisis in the State and the family: Violence against women in Zimbabwe. *African Urban Quarterly, 7* (2&3), 145–162.

UNICEF. (2011). *A situational analysis on the status of women's and children's rights in Zimbabwe, 2005–2010: A call for reducing disparities and improving equity.* Retrieved from http://www.unicef.org/zimbabwe/SitAn_2010-FINAL_FINAL_01-02-2011.pdf

United Nations Human Development Program. (2010). *2010 Human development report.* Retrieved from http://www.beta.undp.org/undp/en/home/presscenter/pressreleases/2010/11/04/undp-launches-2010-human-development-report-analysing-long-term-development-trends.html

United Nations Security Council. (2008, July 11). *Security Council fails to adopt sanctions against Zimbabwe leadership as two permanent members cast negative votes* [press release]. Retrieved from http://www.un.org/News/Press/docs/2008/sc9396.doc.htm

U.S. Department of State Bureau of African Affairs. (2011, October 14). *Zimbabwe: Background notes.* Retrieved from http://www.state.gov/r/pa/ei/bgn/5479.htm

4 Bisexual Identity in a Traditional Culture

A Case Study From Turkey

Senel Poyrazli
Mehmet Eskin

Introduction

In this chapter, a Turkish man's psychosomatic symptoms and his treatment are discussed. However, a word of caution that readers should keep in mind, is that the case story, the practitioner, and the treatment provided in this chapter are not representative of the whole country; therefore, readers should not overgeneralize.

The Authors

The first author, Senel Poyrazli, is a licensed psychologist in the United States and works as an associate professor of counseling psychology at the Pennsylvania State University, Harrisburg campus. Turkish-born, Senel received her undergraduate degree from Hacettepe University, Turkey, in psychological guidance and counseling. She then moved to the United States to attend graduate school. She received her master's degree in counseling psychology from Northeastern University–Boston, and a doctorate degree (American Psychological Association [APA]-accredited) in counseling psychology from the University of Houston, Texas. Senel is a fellow of APA and is actively engaged within different divisions of the APA.

The second author, Dr. Eskin, is a clinical psychologist and works as a full professor at Adnan Menderes University Medical School in Aydin, Turkey. He is a respected clinician and supervisor. He has published several articles and books related to psychological treatment. Dr. Eskin is invited to give seminars throughout Turkey and is one of the key individuals in the country that is interviewed by major newspapers on topics related to psychology. Dr. Eskin's other credentials are presented in the next section.

Senel and Dr. Eskin first met through another professor in Turkey as she was looking for an academician who was well regarded in the community and who could help her write a paper about counseling and psychotherapy in Turkey. After the completion of this project, both authors kept in touch for other things related to their professions.

Throughout this chapter, the second author and the practitioner is referred to as *Dr. Eskin,* rather than by his first name. While it may be more acceptable in some Western cultures, in a Turkish cultural context, it is an extremely disrespectful behavior if somebody at Dr. Eskin's status (i.e., full professor, works as a professional at a medical hospital, etc.) is referred to by his or her first name alone. In addition, the clients and patients who come to seek help at this medical hospital use the word *doctor* or *professor* (*Hocam, Doktor Bey*) to refer to individuals who have the same stature as Dr. Eskin.

The Practitioner

Dr. Eskin received his formal education in Turkey, Norway, and Sweden. He has a bachelor's degree in psychology from the Middle East Technical University (METU), Turkey. He completed graduate work for a master's degree in clinical psychology at METU, and the University of Oslo, Norway. He received his doctoral degree in clinical psychology from Stockholm University, Sweden.

Dr. Eskin is well regarded in Turkey and has several research publications (e.g., Eskin, 2011; Eskin, Ertekin, & Demir, 2008; Eskin, Kaynak-Demir, & Demir, 2005). He is the vice president of the Turkish Psychological Association and actively engages within the community in the delivery of different workshops. He is deemed an effective clinician due to his knowledge base, work experience, and the clinical and communication skills he possesses. He emphasizes and displays a deep respect for clients' integrity, dignity, and self-determination, which positively affects his clients' perception of therapy and the help they are receiving. Dr. Eskin carries a full load of clients. As part of his position at the medical school, he also supervises psychiatry residents and graduate students in clinical psychology. Dr. Eskin is referred new clients by his colleagues or by his previous and current clients. There are times during the year that Dr. Eskin needs to create a waiting list for his new clients who specifically want to see him. However, he is able to convince some of these clients to see the residents and the graduate students he supervises. These clients agree to be seen by another person, knowing that Dr. Eskin will still be involved in the treatment.

In working with his clients, Dr. Eskin follows an existential/humanistic approach that he incorporates into cognitive-behavioral psychotherapy. He refers to the individuals he helps as *clients* as a result of his urging the clients to recognize the power they can have regarding the decisions they make about different aspects of their lives. However, because he works in the psychiatric unit of a medical school, individuals who seek help there are referred to as *patients,* and it is common for a client who seeks help there to see himself or herself as a patient.

Dr. Eskin's therapeutic approach is characterized by an unconditional acceptance and a deep respect for clients' personal decisions and the power they have to lead their lives. He believes that when provided the right therapeutic conditions, individuals have the capability and the potential to find suitable solutions or alternatives related to different aspects of their lives. He considers his main role to be opening up and widening his clients' horizons. In order to achieve this, he uses several cognitive-behavioral techniques and interventions, some of which are Socratic questioning, cognitive restructuring, focusing on beliefs and perceptions as a way to change emotional experiences and behaviors, challenging clients' unhealthy perceptions, using homework assignments, and teaching problem-solving skills. By combining the cognitive-behavioral methods and existential-humanistic methods, Dr. Eskin helps his clients explore who they are, reconnect with themselves, identify their negative perceptions and thoughts especially about themselves, and reconstruct these perceptions and thoughts so that these clients first can accept themselves as they are and then explore what kinds of change should take place in their lives to live a healthier and happier life.

The Case

Mustafa (not client's real name) was a 30-year-old single Muslim man who was college educated. He majored in a discipline that would lead to a career that is considered a traditional career for men. His major is not specified here as a way to further protect his identity. While Mustafa considers himself a believer, he does not practice his religion on a daily basis (e.g., praying five times a day). Physically, Mustafa looks like a masculine man; however, according to the therapist, he has soft speech, frequently sits with his legs crossed much like many women do, and exhibits effeminate mannerisms. Mustafa is his parents' only son and has an older sister who is married. Mustafa lives with both of his parents who are in their 50s; his father is a professional, his mother is a housewife. His father wanted a son, so he was very happy when Mustafa was born.

Mustafa sought help due to intense nausea and burping that prevented him from getting into social situations and seeing others. All medical-physical reasons were ruled out at the department of internal medicine and he was referred for a psychiatric evaluation. While the client's appetite was normal, he did present with a slight disturbance in sleep where he would frequently wake up but then would be able to fall back to sleep. Mustafa denied any suicidal ideation indicating that this was against his religious beliefs and that "only God can take the life he has given."

Besides his parents, another important adult figure in Mustafa's life was his paternal grandfather, who lived close by, frequently involved himself in family affairs, and displayed an authoritarian parenting style. Similar to our client, Mustafa's father was also the only son in the family and the only college-educated sibling. As a result of this, he was highly valued by his family.

Mustafa indicated having a happy childhood. He felt loved by his parents and sister and felt particularly protected and cared for by his mother. Mustafa respected his father greatly and considered him a role model. However, Mustafa also reported some disagreements with his father (e.g., how to run the business or that it is time to get married).

Mustafa experienced his first sexual encounter at the age of 14 with another boy who was 2 to 3 years older than he and lived in the same town as Mustafa. This encounter was a consensual one and Mustafa was the "receiver." He indicated agreeing to this encounter as a result of curiosity. The relationship was purely sexual and took place only one time. There was no emotional or romantic relationship between the two. While Mustafa did not share whether he was satisfied with the encounter, he did express that he is greatly bothered by the possibility that this incident may come out and that he will be shamed in his town. This experience also led to internal conflict due to what he was curious about and how it conflicted with his religious beliefs and the societal values.

Mustafa remembers having more female friends than males in high school. He, however, also reported not having experienced any romantic feelings towards girls during this period. Nonetheless, he considers himself bisexual. He indicated feeling sexually attracted to both genders and reported thinking about both women and men when he sexually fantasized.

Mustafa was academically successful all throughout his primary and secondary education. However, it took him two years to score high enough in the college entrance exam and be placed at a university and a major. In Turkey, college placements are made centrally through the choices presented by the candidate students and based on how well the students score on the exam. One disadvantage of this system is that the student is not allowed to switch majors without some rather stiff consequences. In order to study in a different major, the student must again take the competitive college entrance test that is offered only once a year. When Mustafa was placed at a university, even though he did not like his major (a major that would lead to a traditionally male career), he followed his father's request and enrolled. When he was in his junior year, he took the entrance exam again and was placed into another major, which too led to a traditionally male career. His family was supportive of his career change; Mustafa enrolled and graduated with his college degree. Despite his degree, Mustafa does not practice his profession. He instead owns and operates a retail store. The decision to enter into a different line of work, however, is not an uncommon one. As Mustafa is the only son, he was expected to move back home after his college education and live with and take care of his parents. He lived in a small town where it was extremely difficult to find a job related to his college education. To be able to stay with his parents and fulfill cultural expectations, he opened a retail store and reported being happy with his work.

The Context

Turkey is situated in southeastern Europe and western Asia with land in both continents and strategically positioned within the Middle East. The country is surrounded by the Mediterranean Sea, the Aegean Sea, and the Black Sea, and neighbors by land the countries of Greece, Bulgaria, Armenia, Azerbaijan, Georgia, Iran, Iraq, and Syria. The population is 78 million and the majority of the population is Muslim (Central Intelligence Agency, 2011).

Considering the presenting problems for Mustafa, it is important to discuss two particular contextual conditions in Turkey: prejudice and discrimination towards lesbian, gay, bisexual, and transgendered (LGBT) individuals, and gender role socialization and expectations.

Parents in Turkey engage in several methods to show that being gay is not acceptable. To change or oppress their nonheterosexual child, parents may engage in behaviors such as "taking [the child] to psychiatrists to provide treatment, expelling him/her from home, and punishing him/her by threats, beating, and by limiting social support" (Oksal, 2008, p. 514). Witnessing these types of oppressions and exclusions likely make Turkish LGBT persons fear that they would lose their family's support and be subjected to similar treatments if they were to come out to their families.

Discrimination towards LGBT groups both in law and practice is present in Turkey (Amnesty International, 2011). These deeply rooted negative attitudes and prejudice towards LGBT groups partly stem from the religion of Islam, which characterizes homosexuality as sin. In its 2010 annual report, Amnesty International presents several cases where, for example, a gay man was killed by his father (honor killing), but the father was not charged with the crime right away despite the evidence. In another case, prosecutors tried to close down several organizations supporting LGBT groups based on the claim that they encouraged individuals to have a nonheterosexual orientation.

In addition to Amnesty International, The U.S. Department of State (2011) also reports that LGBT individuals in Turkey face problems as a result of their sexual orientation and gender identity. These individuals are frequently discriminated against by others and also by the government officials and law enforcement groups. Two government entities, the Directorate of Religious Affairs and the State Ministry in Charge of Women and Family Affairs, deemed homosexuality as unacceptable and as a disease that needs to be treated. The 2010 Human Rights Report (U.S. Department of State, 2011) indicates that these types of statements provoke further discrimination by ordinary people onto LGBT individuals. The report further indicates that the government issued warnings to TV stations for including gay couples in their shows and for making homosexuality look normal and acceptable. The report also presents cases where openly LGBT individuals have been fired from their jobs or have been harassed or beaten by the police officers for being openly gay. Just like the report indicates, unfortunately there are many cases where LGBT individuals have lost their jobs. In a prominent case that made the newspapers, a gay elementary school teacher was fired from his job for having homosexual relations with men (Basaran, 2010). This teacher hid his sexual identity from the community he lived in and from his coworkers for fear of discrimination. However, a male individual who came to learn the teacher's sexual identity made an effort to solicit him sexually. When the teacher refused, this individual retaliated by telling the community that the teacher was gay. The teacher, subsequently, was fired from his job. He has exhausted all of the legal channels in Turkey, including the Supreme Court. He currently has a case pending against the Turkish government with the European Court of Human Rights (ECHR). He hopes that the ECHR will help him get his job back.

Despite these reports of discriminatory behaviors, there are many developments that follow an orientation toward fairness in work and school settings, the quelling of violence against "outed" LGBT people, and even an increase in organized groups meeting in support of their identities. Many LGBT groups in Turkey try to consistently organize, make their voices heard, and reduce prejudice and discrimination against themselves. The Human Rights Report (U.S. Department of State, 2011) discusses college student groups who tried to get permission from their college presidents to form an LGBT club on their campuses. Some of these attempts have been successful. Another positive development is that a court in a large city dismissed a decision to close one of the LGBT rights associations, the Black Pink Triangle. The court's ruling in favor of the association may have been a result of Turkey's attempt to get in to the European Union (EU) which demanded that human rights be improved in Turkey before Turkey's application to get into the EU is considered. Some of these positive developments are also portrayed in the media. Many TV channels and shows discuss and present issues related to the LGBT groups. Several LGBT organizations offer workshops, hold protests, or arrange campaigns with different themes such as "You are neither wrong nor alone!" ("*Ne yanlış, ne de yalnızsınız!*") to provide support for the LGBT individuals and to educate the public. Moreover, Turkish researchers are increasingly studying LGBT issues and disseminating their findings through conference presentations or journal article publications (e.g., Bereket & Adam, 2006; Cirakoglu, 2006; Eskin, Kaynak-Demir, & Demir, 2005; Gelbal & Duyan, 2006; Oksal, 2008). These positive developments help, for example, more and more gays to "incorporate their homosexual behavior into their sense of self and comfortably identify themselves under the *gey* label as a social identity" (Bereket & Adam, 2006, p. 132). These developments also help more and more individuals to be tolerant of LGBT persons and even be more accepting of them.

There are very few publications related to bisexual individuals in a Turkish context. As a result, information was drawn from the literature about Turkish gay and lesbians to help readers understand the possible experiences of a bisexual Turkish person.

In relation to gender role socialization and expectations, Turkish culture tends to be relatively traditional. Turkish parents tend to expect traditional gender roles from their children and socialize their children based on cultural stereotypes related to how women and men should feel, behave, and dress (Oksal, 2008). Sons are expected to continue the family name, which requires having male children. In Turkish law, a newborn can have only one last name and that has to be the father's last name. Sons are also expected to care for their parents in their elder years (Kagitcibasi, 1994); having a wife makes it easier for this to happen as day-to-day care is expected to come from women. Men are pressured to find a woman to marry and have children (Bereket & Adam, 2006), especially after completing their mandatory military service. As a result of this pressure, many gay or bisexual men concede to the pressure and marry women.

In comparison to girls, the Turkish culture allows more independence for boys during childhood; however, even for boys, strong independence is not encouraged (Kagitcibasi & Sunar, 1992). In fact, many adult sons are expected to strongly consider or follow their parents' wishes when making decisions and choices about their lives, and in some cases, these individuals sacrifice their own goals for the goals set for them by their parents (Poyrazli, 2003). As a result of this gender role socialization and traditional aspect of the culture, it is extremely hard for LGBT individuals to share their sexual orientation and identity with their parents or families despite the many positive developments that have taken place within the Turkish society.

The Treatment

Mustafa received a nine-session treatment based on an existential-humanistic framework incorporated into cognitive-behavioral approaches. During the intake, Mustafa focused on his burping and nausea, and believed they were based on medical reasons that needed to be explored through additional tests. In this first session, he shared that he made wrong choices in his life and was regretful; however, he hesitated to indicate what these wrong choices were. Considering that this was the first session and sensing his hesitancy to speak about these choices, Dr. Eskin left it to another session to explore what these "wrong choices" were.

In order to find out what psychological reasons caused these psychosomatic symptoms, Mustafa was asked to keep a record of when, where, and what time these symptoms occurred, whether he was with anybody, and what thoughts were going through his mind right before and after the symptoms occurred. He kept this record every day for about three weeks. Between the first and second sessions, Mustafa also completed a set of questionnaires to help Dr. Eskin further assess Mustafa's psychological experiences. He scored 22 on the Beck Depression Inventory and 17 on the Beck Anxiety Inventory, indicating mild depression and anxiety. His scores on an identity measure specifically developed for Turkish individuals (Sense of Identity Assessment Form; *Kimlik Duygusu Değerlendirme Aracı*) indicated evidence that he was confused about his overall identity. An evaluation of his answers on the Rotter Sentence Completion Test indicated that Mustafa sometimes felt weak and powerless. The biggest fear he had was losing his loved ones. He viewed others as unloving, uncaring, unsupportive, unemotional, and as people who cannot be trusted. He felt angry at people for being overly involved in others' lives. He experienced confusion and difficulty in concentration. He seemed unhappy and in search of different experiences in his life. It bothered him that he was not content and happy with his life. His other answers on the test indicated that he felt attracted to those of his gender, felt remorse about his first sexual encounter with the boy in his town, and was concerned that this experience may haunt him. Mustafa believed he took the wrong sexual road and hated himself for not being able to get rid of his same-sex attraction.

Mustafa was clearly experiencing an internal conflict. He wanted to please his family and do the right things, but his attraction to men did not allow that to happen. In order to resolve this internal conflict, he felt that he either needed to reject his bisexual identity or his family and his culture. Rejecting himself seemed to be the easier choice. Before coming to counseling, he accepted his family's and relatives' attempts to find him a girl to marry. For example, he visited different homes with his parents where there would be a girl that was ready for marriage or he agreed to meet with potential girls for coffee to see if they would click together.

Discussions, starting with the second session, revealed that Mustafa's sexual experiences had mostly been with men. He also indicated having limited sexual experience with women. Mustafa shared with Dr. Eskin that when he had sexual fantasies, watched or looked at porn, or masturbated, he thought about both men and women. When Dr. Eskin asked him what he thought his sexual orientation was, Mustafa indicated seeing himself as bisexual. In Turkish culture, homosexuality or bisexuality is considered a sexual activity rather than an orientation, which leads individuals to place an emphasis on their sexual activity and who they feel closer to sexually (Bereket & Adam, 2006). Knowing this emphasis and wanting to help the client have a better understanding of what sexual orientation is, Dr. Eskin also explored which gender Mustafa felt close to emotionally and with whom Mustafa fell in love in the past. From his answers, it seemed that Mustafa mostly felt emotionally and romantically close to men, while he also reported a few women with whom he was romantically involved. He fell in love only once, with a man, when he was in college. However, there was no relationship, only strong feelings from Mustafa that were not shared with the man. Mustafa also reported that through an online portal, he found men to date and to have "hook-ups." He traveled out of town away from home for these mostly sexual activities with other men so that people in his town did not find out that he was bisexual. Mustafa, however, expressed dissatisfaction that the men he had been with "only wanted sex" and that he yearned for a "romantic and close" relationship. In other words, while hooking up with other men interested in men seemed relatively easy to do, the task of finding romantic partners was more difficult for Mustafa.

When Mustafa shared his sexual encounters, Dr. Eskin provided psychoeducational information about how to protect himself against sexually transmitted infections. Dr. Eskin provides this information as part of his routine work with all of his sexually active clients. Mustafa appreciated the information and indicated practicing safe sex.

It is important to discuss the therapeutic conditions that may have helped Mustafa to move from a "my symptoms are medical based" point of view in the first session to a "my symptoms are psychosomatic and related to my bisexualism" point of view in the subsequent sessions. Dr. Eskin is deemed as a good listener by his colleagues and clients. As part of the first and second sessions, he gives his clients an opportunity to tell their stories. He engages in reflective listening, often paraphrasing or summarizing what the client is saying, reflecting the client's emotions, and asking clarifying questions. The most common communication style practiced by people in the Turkish culture is based on asking questions and giving advice, and anecdotally, it is safe for the authors to conclude that individuals rarely have the feeling that they are fully listened to and heard by others. As a result, Dr. Eskin's reflective style pleases his clients from the very beginning and helps them experience relief from telling their story without being interrupted, questioned, or being presented with solutions or advice regarding how they should deal with their problems. His clients often indicate to Dr. Eskin that they feel understood by him and that they can tell that he knows what they are going through. Another point Dr. Eskin covers in the first session is the fact that, with the exception of some limits, the counseling and therapy process is a confidential process and what the client shares is not repeated. He also informs the clients that while he will have several questions that he will ask, the clients are free not to answer certain questions if they do not wish to do so. Dr. Eskin shares this information as a way to recognize clients' power and also to help them realize that they have the power to make certain choices in their lives. As a result, this information giving and creation of certain therapeutic conditions played a role in Mustafa trusting Dr. Eskin and feeling comfortable to discuss his bisexuality and consider his sexual orientation as a reason for his psychosomatic symptoms.

At the same time, while he considered himself as bisexual, Mustafa also felt conflicted that this orientation was against his religious, Muslim beliefs. He felt greatly bothered about his orientation and viewed bisexualism as unacceptable. Mustafa indicated during therapy that he considered any type of homosexuality as sick and that he wanted Dr. Eskin to show him ways to get rid of his same-sex attraction. Dr. Eskin concluded that this type of desire for curing his homosexuality was directly in line with Turkish society's negative attitudes towards any type of homosexual feeling or activity and the perception that heterosexuality is the only healthy orientation. Knowing about the society's attitudes and having a sexual orientation that is not heterosexual can lead individuals to experience internal conflict and confusion. Dr. Eskin also concluded that Mustafa was suffering from internalized homophobia. Later in the therapy process, Dr. Eskin shared with Mustafa that both biological and psychological factors are involved in the development of sexual orientation (Bem, 1996; Bem, 2000; James, 2005; Rahman & Wilson, 2003) and discussed internalized homophobia with him. He informed Mustafa that people who experience internalized homophobia display hatred towards themselves for having a nonheterosexual orientation and that they display strong rejection of their identity so that they are not in conflict with the society and in Mustafa's case, also with their religious beliefs. Mustafa felt enlightened by this information and was surprised how well this concept explained his internal conflict. He expressed relief as a result of the new perspective he had gained; he was better able to understand why he had so many negative feelings towards himself and his orientation.

Dr. Eskin and Mustafa analyzed the weekly records he kept and tried to track his psychosomatic symptoms. It was apparent that nausea and burping occurred when Mustafa was in the shower and also when he was with his family members. By using this weekly record, Dr. Eskin explored whether these psychosomatic symptoms were related to the client being bisexual. Mustafa, in the therapy process, found this explanation to be a reasonable one. Through the help Dr. Eskin provided, Mustafa came to the conclusion that there were several reasons for why and where these symptoms were taking place. When he saw himself naked in the shower, his body reminded him of men with whom he had sex. Seeing himself naked also reminded him of the same-sex attraction he had, awakened his internalized homophobia, and he started feeling nauseated and burped. Dr. Eskin's conclusion was that Mustafa was experiencing internal conflict due to his sexual orientation being in contradiction with what the Turkish society viewed as normal and acceptable. In this conflict, the society won: Mustafa felt helpless and powerless, and as a result, his psychosomatic symptoms would take place. From a humanistic/existential perspective, Mustafa's distress stemmed from his urges to self-actualize and be himself. However, the cultural context that he lived in was preventing him from self-actualizing.

Mustafa also gained insight that the reason his symptoms occurred in his family's presence was related to the Turkish society's and his family's expectations for him. The culture expected that somebody of Mustafa's age who completed his education and military service and had employment would get married and have children. His parents wanted to have grandchildren. If such a son doesn't consider getting married, the situation creates confusion for the parents, other relatives, friends, and even neighbors who frequently believe they have the right to get involved in their neighbors' lives. During the therapy sessions, Mustafa shared that his family was pressuring him to get married and that they were "bride shopping." In Turkish culture, if a person is deemed ready to be married and this person has not yet identified an individual to marry, the family members and other relatives take it upon themselves to find suitable prospects and present these possibilities to the person. When Mustafa was with his family members, they brought up the topic of marriage and said things like "when are you going to get married," "time is running out," or "when are we going to have grandchildren." On the other hand, Mustafa knew that coming out to his family was "out of the question" and that if his family knew that he was bisexual, it would turn his "world upside down." As a result, when he was with his family, Mustafa was put in a situation to face his bisexuality and felt like he was a disappointment, which in turn triggered his nausea and burping.

Evaluation of Treatment

Focusing on his internal conflict and the homophobic nature of the Turkish culture helped Mustafa experience relief. Mustafa came to the conclusion that if he lived in a more accepting culture, he would be happy with his sexual orientation. In addition, information giving was used as a way to further educate him about the difficulties he experienced within the Turkish culture while also sharing with him that the contemporary psychiatry and psychology in Turkey and elsewhere do not regard homosexuality and bisexualism as abnormal. These psycho-educational discussions gradually reduced the nausea and burping Mustafa experienced.

At the end of the ninth session, Mustafa's psychosomatic symptoms were almost nonexistent. Both the client and Dr. Eskin decided it was time to terminate treatment. Dr. Eskin informed Mustafa that he was welcome to make an appointment in the future if the intensity and frequency of his symptoms worsened or if he needed to receive counseling or therapy for a different reason. About eight or nine months after the termination session, Dr. Eskin ran into Mustafa in a parking lot. Dr. Eskin does not acknowledge his clients out in public first, so that the clients' confidentiality is protected. However, he does briefly chat with his clients if they initiate the conversation first. In this incident, Mustafa approached Dr. Eskin and was very happy to see him. He told Dr. Eskin that his nausea and burping had completely disappeared. He thanked Dr. Eskin again for the help he had provided.

During counseling, Dr. Eskin made the observation that after Mustafa admitted to his sexual orientation, the topics for every following session centered on bisexuality, Mustafa's internal conflict, and his family's pressures to marry which also conflicted with his sexual orientation. Mustafa perhaps saw his sessions as a safe haven where he could talk about the things he could not talk with others outside. Sharing his fears, pent-up emotions, pressures he felt, and anxiety about his sexual orientation helped him experience relief, which then led to a better understanding of what he was experiencing and how those experiences were related to the culture in which he lived. Cognitive restructuring was proven to be a very useful technique to help Mustafa gain new perspectives and understanding in the therapy process. For example, in one of the sessions Dr. Eskin asked Mustafa to indicate at what percentage he thought sexuality contributed to a person's whole identity and life. Mustafa's response was "30 to 35%." Dr. Eskin then asked how much Mustafa thought sexuality contributed to his own identity and life. Mustafa was surprised to realize that his "whole" identity and life seemed to have been made up of sexuality and that he was preoccupied with his sexuality. During and after the termination of the process, Dr. Eskin wondered whether Mustafa used the term *bisexualism* as a way to help himself escape from the more negative stigma associated with being *gay*. Many gay individuals introduce themselves as bisexuals to reduce the likelihood of being rejected. In Turkish culture, for a person even to admit he or she is bisexual is quite a risk. As a result, Dr. Eskin did not want to put Mustafa in a more uncomfortable position by exploring whether he might be gay. Dr. Eskin was able to discuss the culture, society's expectations, pressures Mustafa was facing, and how all of these factors were contributing to Mustafa's symptoms by focusing on his bisexual identity. However, Dr. Eskin wondered if Mustafa was gay, not bisexual, and whether he would give in to society's pressure and marry a woman. If this ever becomes the case, Mustafa may experience similar psychosomatic symptoms and may decide to come back for more counseling and therapy.

The authors believe that it may have been an advantage for Mustafa to have a heterosexual psychologist. Mustafa knew that Dr. Eskin was married to a woman and had a family and as a result, lived a heterosexual life.

He heard about this before coming to see Dr. Eskin. In addition, Dr. Eskin wears a gold ring in his left hand, which indicates that he is married and by implication, heterosexual.

Mustafa lives in an extremely heterosexist culture. Having a heterosexual helper who presented homosexuality and bisexuality as normal may have helped Mustafa to have an easier time exploring and honoring his sexual identity. The authors also believe that having a psychologist who was older than he was may have further benefited him. In Turkish culture, elders' perception and opinions are important. Mustafa was surrounded by people who were older than him (e.g., his parents, grandfather, etc.) who were trying to show him the "right way," which was to get married and to have children. Dr. Eskin, who is 15 years older than Mustafa, understood and normalized Mustafa's sexual orientation and his ambivalence towards marriage. Furthermore, having a male psychologist may have also helped Mustafa. Homophobia in Turkish culture is perpetrated more by men than women, at least as revealed openly and violently. Harassment, rape, and honor killing type of behaviors towards LGBT persons are almost always carried out by men. Therefore, Dr. Eskin embracing Mustafa's sexual orientation may have helped Mustafa see that some men will accept, acknowledge, and respect him for his sexual orientation.

While Mustafa experienced relief and seemed to have accepted his bisexualism at the end of the counseling process, he is still likely to continue experiencing internal conflict as it would not be easy for anybody to erase or forget cultural messages he has been given related to what is an acceptable sexual orientation. He also will not be able to forget memories and oppressive behaviors he has been subjected to as a result of his sexual orientation. Therefore, he will continue experiencing periodic conflicts especially when he remembers the exclusion, prejudice, intolerance, and oppression he faced and what his culture deems as healthy and unhealthy sexual orientation.

A limitation of the counseling process Mustafa received was that it focused on symptom relief. When his psychosomatic symptoms were almost nonexistent and the client thought that the goal of relieving these symptoms was achieved, Dr. Eskin agreed to termination. However, Dr. Eskin also believes that Mustafa's treatment may be only the beginning of a larger counseling process that still needs to take place. If Mustafa decides to come back to see Dr. Eskin, the following are some additional goals to consider:

1. Further exploring Mustafa's sexual identity to see if he is bisexual or gay. The number of options Mustafa could have will depend on exploring his identity. If he is bisexual, he may be able to enter into a heterosexual relationship that he knows will please his family. However, if he is gay, this option may be much more difficult for him to consider.

2. Expanding Mustafa's social support system in a way that he could have people who embrace him fully for his sexual orientation. Even though he lives in a small, close-knit town and establishing an LGBT-friendly support system may not be an option, he could still create this social support system through joining online support groups.

3. Finding better ways to balance his individual needs and the society's and his family's expectations that he should get married.

4. Addressing religion and helping him find ways to be at peace with his religion and sexual orientation. Mustafa is Muslim and following his religious beliefs, he considers homosexuality as sin. He needs to explore to see whether or not he needs to make a decision to practice more in consort with his religious beliefs and perhaps not follow his romantic attraction to men. In addition, in a nonjudgmental therapy environment, Mustafa should also explore whether or not he can embrace his sexual identity and religious beliefs together in harmony, and if not, which one he should consider being more important.

5. Helping him realize that his whole identity is more than his sexual identity; that he has other things such as his work, career, personality, religion, social relationships, and so on, that are a part of his identity in addition to his sexual orientation.

Conclusion

Some mental health professionals, following an individual paradigm, may believe that Mustafa should accept his sexual identity in its totality and follow his individual goals even if that involves some extreme measures such as rejecting his family or culture. The authors, however, argue a different point: For clients like Mustafa who are from a more collectivistic and traditional culture as compared to some of the western cultures, an approach where the client is helped to find ways to balance his or her needs and goals with cultural expectations will lead to a more effective treatment outcome and better mental health for the client.

References

Amnesty International. (2011). *2010 Annual report for Turkey*. Retrieved from http://www.amnestyusa.org/annualreport.php?id=ar&yr=2010&c=TUR

Basaran, E. (2010, December 5). Escinsel ilahiyatci sinifini geri istiyor. *Radikal*. Retrieved from http://www.radikal.com.tr/Default.aspx?aType=RadikalYazar&Date=5.12.2010&ArticleID=1031426

Bem, D. J. (1996). Exotic becomes erotic: A developmental theory of sexual orientation. *Psychological Review, 103,* 320–335.

Bem, D. J. (2000). Exotic becomes erotic: Interpreting the biological correlates of sexual orientation. *Archives of Sexual Behavior, 29,* 531–548.

Bereket, T., & Adam, B. D. (2006). The emergence of gay identities in contemporary Turkey. *Sexualities, 9,* 131–151.

Central Intelligence Agency. (2011). *The world factbook: Turkey.* Retrieved from https://www.cia.gov/library/publications/the-world-factbook/geos/tu.html

Cirakoglu, O. C. (2006). Perception of homosexuality among Turkish university students: The roles of labels, gender, and prior contact. *The Journal of Social Psychology, 146,* 293–305.

Eskin, M. (2011). Türk gençlerinde cinsel yönelim çalışmaları [Studies related to sexual orientation among the Turkish youth]. In M. Eskin, C. Dereboy, H. Harlak & F. Dereboy, (Eds.). *Türkiye'de Gençlik: Ne biliyoruz? Ne bilmiyoruz? [Youth in Turkey: What do we know? What do we not know?].* Manuscript submitted for publication. Ankara, Turkey: Hekimler Yayın Birliği Yayınları.

Eskin, M., Ertekin, K., & Demir, H. (2008). Efficacy of a problem-solving therapy for depression and suicide potential in adolescents and young adults. *Cognitive Therapy and Research, 32,* 227–245.

Eskin, M., Kaynak-Demir, H., & Demir, S. (2005). Same-sex orientation, childhood sexual abuse, and suicidal behavior in university students in Turkey. *Archives of Sexual Behavior, 34,* 185–195.

Gelbal, S., & Duyan, V. (2006). Attitudes of university students toward lesbians and gay men in Turkey. *Sex Roles, 55,* 573–579.

James, W. H. (2005). Biological and psychosocial determinants of male and female human sexual orientation. *Journal of Biosocial Science, 37,* 555–567.

Kagitcibasi, C. (1994). Psychology in Turkey. *International Journal of Psychology, 26,* 729–738.

Kagitcibasi, C., & Sunar, D. (1992). Family and socialization in Turkey. In J. L. Raopnarine & D. B. Carter (Eds.), *Parent-child socialization in diverse cultures* (pp. 75–88). Norwood, NJ: Ablex.

Oksal, A. (2008). Turkish family members' attitudes toward lesbians and gay men. *Sex Roles, 58,* 514–525.

Poyrazli, S. (2003). Validity of Rogerian Therapy in Turkish culture: A cross-cultural perspective. *Journal of Humanistic Counseling, Education, and Development, 42,* 107–115.

Rahman, Q., & Wilson, G. D. (2003). Born gay? The psychobiology of human sexual orientation. *Personality and Individual Differences, 34,* 1337–1382.

U.S. Department of State. (2011). *2010 Human rights report: Turkey.* Retrieved from: http://www.state.gov/g/drl/rls/hrrpt/2010/eur/154455.htm

5 Case Study of a Female Patient With Anxiety Disorder and Depression

Psychotherapy Within a Lebanese Cultural Framework

Brigitte Khoury

_____ **Introduction of the Author**

I, Brigitte Khoury, am from Lebanon, was born in Paris, France, and was raised in Beirut. In 1992, I went to pursue my PhD in California, United States, and stayed there until 1997 when I ended my postdoctorate fellowship. Upon my return to Beirut, Lebanon, I started working as a faculty member at the psychiatry department at the American University of Beirut Medical Center (AUB-MC) and have been there since. Back then, I was the first and only clinical psychologist in the department and in the faculty ranks in the medical school. Later on, I was the founding president of the Lebanese Psychological Association, which played a major role in raising the awareness of the public about mental health issues, initiated the drafting of rules and regulations of practice with governmental bodies, and pulled together the majority of Lebanese psychologists into a network. It is worth noting that, in Lebanon, the number of psychologists per

The author would like to thank Ms. Yasmine Fayad who contributed to the writing of this chapter.

100,000 population is low (approximately 0.6) and efforts to gather these professionals and increase their cooperation are crucial to improve mental health care and better meet the needs of the Lebanese population (World Health Organization, 2005).

I was trained in cognitive-behavioral therapy (Beck, 1995) and interpersonal therapy (Teyber, 2006), which I see as valuable in my work with most Lebanese clients. I also use other methods that better fit the Lebanese culture. Some of these methods include advice giving, supportive counseling, and family therapy and techniques (Rasheed, Rasheed, & Marley, 2011). I freely incorporate religion and spiritual references in the helping process based on the belief system of clients who are pious, whether Christians or Muslims. I particularly favor supportive counseling, which enhances the functioning of patients by helping them develop the means to resolve their own problems and improve their coping skills (Poulin, 2009).

The Practitioner

Given that I am working in a hospital, most of the labels used are influenced by the medical context. Hence, *clients* are referred to as *patients*, thus facilitating the communication with other medical professionals and referral sources from inside the hospital or outside the hospital. Diagnostic labels, on the other hand, are carefully dealt with and used differently when communicating with patients and families than with colleagues in the mental health profession. In an American institution where all faculty members are trained in the United States, the *Diagnostic and Statistical Manual,* Fourth Edition (*DSM-IV-TR*) is commonly used to diagnose patients and guide treatment. The manual serves as a means of communication with other health care professionals, hence providing them with a common vernacular.

However, the use of these diagnostic labels when communicating with patients and family members depends on their exposure to Western-based education. Other factors related to patient or family characteristics are also taken into consideration in deciding how certain information is disclosed. This is especially true when the diagnosis applied to the patient is highly stigmatized in the culture. Certainly, I sometimes withhold explicit information about the diagnosis from families and even the patients if it risks hindering or sabotaging the therapeutic process. For instance, it would be overwhelming, if not crushing, for some patients to know that they have a personality disorder. Hence, such information is reframed and conveyed in a less pathologizing way in order not to de-motivate patients or discourage them from coming to therapy.

Whether or not a diagnostic label is disclosed, I always educate my patients about their disorder to empower them while at the same time show my acceptance of and sensitivity to their conception of mental illness. The cultural understanding of the psychological problem in the Lebanese context may be quite different from the way it is described in the *DSM*. Patients and their families use different expressions to describe mental illness such as "nerves are tired" (in dialectical Arabic, "أعصاب تعبيني") and "nervous breakdown" (in dialectical Arabic, "انهيار عصبي") and different explanations to define its causes such as "she was under pressure from work and family so she collapsed" or "she had problems with her husband and so her nerves could not take it anymore."

It is worth noting that patients in this cultural context tend to describe mental illness in somatic terms as illustrated by the expression of "nerves are tired," which based on its literal meaning, is more indicative of a physical rather than a psychological illness. In my practice, I am aware of the patients' tendency to express their distress through somatic metaphors and mindful of the psychological meanings often carried by such expressions. In addition to being sensitive to the language used to describe mental illness, I also avoid challenging sociocultural beliefs related to the etiology of the psychological disorder even when they stand in sharp contrast to a Western biomedical model. For example, some patients tend to attribute psychological disturbance to supernatural factors such as the evil eye and, in such situations, I refrain from judgment and try to understand the patient in his or her sociocultural context.

Based on anecdotal evidence gathered from patients, the main criteria for determining the competence of mental health professionals in Lebanon, other than working in a well-known institution such as the AUB-MC, are the professionals' ability to ensure confidentiality and achieve success with other patients.

In Lebanon, a health professional is deemed competent when, from word of mouth, different people talk about his or her success with a friend or family member. This is no exception with psychology. Hence, many individuals are referred to therapy by other patients or their family members who had a positive experience with me and would recommend me to others. They would come in and say to me, "My friend so and so, or neighbor, or aunt came to you and you helped him or her a lot, so I wanted also to come over and ask you to solve my problems." Based on my patients' feedback, I realized that being a straightforward yet empowering therapist helped many patients to improve. These patients were thankful for being helped to believe in themselves, to minimize their fears, and to move to real action. Feedback from patients such as "I am more confident," "I don't feel stuck anymore," and "I feel stronger" frequently encourage new patients to seek therapy. Another encouraging factor is the use of cognitive-behavioral therapy. Directive and guided techniques are agreeable to people because they provide something to do, to think of, or to apply in the real world. Thus, patients feel that therapy teaches them new coping skills, hence encouraging them to feel its effects concretely.

Confidentiality is still a major issue to consider when seeking mental health help in Lebanon. Patients and their families fear being stigmatized due to the mental illness. Many patients are concerned about being labeled mentally ill and hence, perceived as incompetent, which could lead to being mocked and taken advantage of. Therefore, being able to access confidential services, where patients' privacy is respected, is a major attraction to Lebanese patients and families. Respecting confidentiality is one of the main conditions of offering proper mental health services according to the American Psychological Association's (APA) ethical guidelines (APA, 2002) as well as AUB-MC standards of practice. I always reassure my patients about their right to confidentiality, yet am very clear from the outset of therapy about its limits. In addition, when family members call me on the phone to discuss a patient, without indicating whether the person in question is my patient, I explain the limits of confidentiality and encourage the family to talk to the patient directly. I also inform them that I allow family members to come with the patient to one of the sessions to discuss their concern. This is a good way to maintain confidentiality while also engage the family in the treatment.

Although I was trained and licensed as a clinical psychologist in the United States, I realized as soon as I started working in Lebanon that to succeed in this context many skills and theories taught in the West had to be adjusted to the local culture. One of my first experiences as a cognitive-behavior therapist was to give homework to a patient tapping into his negative thinking patterns. The patient did not take it seriously and thought that I was treating him like a child and being insensitive to his pain. He did not do the homework but later on understood the importance of negative perceptions and how changing them helped him. However, instead of doing the homework with paper and pencil, he and I talked about it in the session, which made him feel validated and respected. Based on this experience, I started educating my patients about the use of homework assignments and why they are very valuable to the therapy process. I also explored whether patients felt comfortable with reporting on their homework in a written way or if they preferred to provide a verbal report. I realized that the theory may apply but often the practical aspects of it may not, hence it had to be adjusted to the culture. Therefore, I had to let go of many techniques which I found inapplicable to the culture as well as pick up new skills and ways of treatment that I had not learned in my Western training. For example, I came to learn the importance of the family for Lebanese patients. Lebanese therapists do not involve only the individual in the treatment but also the family, which becomes one of the most important allies for the therapy to succeed. If the therapist does not involve the family in the treatment process and discuss the individual's improvement, the family may convince the individual to discontinue his or her treatment or to switch therapists. I should also note that there are times when the family members are causing harm to the patient and their involvement in the treatment is not desired by the patient nor is it clinically advised.

There are many ways Lebanese families insert their cultural rights to get involved and make it known to the therapist that they want to contribute to the treatment. For example, they may show up to the session with the patient, demand to come into the room with the patient, want to talk to the therapist after or before the patient's session, call the therapist to ask questions, or simply show up at the therapist's office at a different time than the patient's scheduled session to discuss the patient and his or her treatment. When the patient wants his or her family to be involved in the therapy process and the family is willing to do so, I allow this to happen. Sometimes, when I meet with family members alone, the conversation ends up being about them and their stress rather than the patient's condition. When this happens, I consistently shift the focus back to the patient gently but firmly and try to relate the information provided by the family member to the treatment and the patient's well-being. However, if it is clear that a family member also needs help, I refer him or her to be seen by one of my colleagues.

Although it is quite challenging to deal with the family in addition to the patient, the impact of the context on individuals' well-being should not be overlooked in a culture where individuals do not exist independently of others (Dwairy, 2006; Harb & Smith, 2008). Involving the family in the patient's treatment contributes to the effectiveness of therapy in many ways. It may increase compliance and emotional support or help identify culturally appropriate ways to resolve intrafamilial conflicts.

The Case

Mona is a 45-year-old married Lebanese Christian female, who worked in a company as an administrator for the past three years. She lives with her husband of 22 years and their two children, a boy who is 17 and a girl who is 20 years old. She was referred to me by a psychiatrist who had provided medication evaluation for anxiety and depression. In addition to the medication treatment, the psychiatrist wanted Mona to receive psychotherapy treatment.

Mona came in for the first time with her mother, an elderly woman who answered all the questions on her behalf, leaving very little room for Mona to speak. This method of communication is quite common in the Lebanese culture. Older family members take it upon themselves to answer questions about the patient regardless of the patient's age. After allowing the mother to fulfill her cultural role by answering some of the questions on behalf of the patient, I asked the mother to wait in the lobby so that the second part of the intake that involved me being alone with the patient could be accomplished. The mother understood that I needed to spend time alone with her daughter during the treatment. Mona seemed uncomfortable to be alone. She may have liked her mother answering the questions since this made it easier for her to be interviewed. When seen alone, Mona reported her inability to face problems and getting easily overwhelmed and anxious, which made her feel down. Her sleep and appetite were poor. She cried often over her helplessness and seemed to catastrophize her situation. She had poor self-esteem and always feared losing her job, although her boss was happy with her performance. Mona worried that her depression and anxiety, which increased her need for time-off, would eventually lead to her being fired from work. She asked for a one-week sick leave from work when she came to see me and worried that she may need more time off since she felt unable to handle her responsibilities at work. We discussed the possibility of her taking more time off in order to work on herself and feel better and then going back gradually, possibly part-time initially before going back full-time. Mona agreed to the plan and talked to her boss, who agreed to the arrangement. It was clear that she was liked at work and her boss thought highly of her, so he gave her the time she needed. This relieved Mona from an immense source of pressure and worry.

Mona reported that her symptoms started three months earlier and she could no longer take care of her household or do any of the necessary chores. Hence, she moved in with her parents who lived about 20 minutes away, leaving her husband behind to take care of the children and the house. This arrangement was against the social expectations of her role as a wife, mother, and homemaker, whose main task is to care for her household and her nuclear family. Many proverbs illustrate this role for women such as "the mother is the one who raises the children" (in dialectical Arabic "بتربى الأم,") and "the mother pulls together the family" (in dialectical Arabic "الام بتلم"), and "the woman builds the home" (in dialectical Arabic "الام بتعمر البيت"). These expectations created more distress for Mona who saw herself failing in her role towards her family and her community. The explanation given was that "her nerves were tired" and she needed to rest and relax at her parents' house. The understanding, of course, was that once feeling better she would return to her own family and resume her roles of wife and mother.

A major stressor Mona mentioned was related to her teenage son being in conflict with his father, who Mona believed did not understand the son. Mona's husband often complained that the son did not care about schoolwork and underachieved, that he was always out of the house with his friends, that he stayed up late, and that he always went out without them knowing where he was. He once caught the son smoking and that made him feel enraged and he kicked the son out of the house. That night the son stayed at a friend's house and, per Mona's statement, had it not been for Mona begging him the next day to come back home, he would not have. Mona often had to defend her son from the father's verbal abuse and raised voice. Often, her husband complained about their son to her and blamed her for not setting the proper limits and rules for him. Other times, the son would complain to her about the father and threaten to leave home. Several times she fought with her husband and defended the son and also blamed the husband for their son being away most of the time and not wanting to stay home. Being in the middle between them affected Mona tremendously and contributed to her feeling increasingly helpless, depressed, and anxious. She described herself as a "worrier" over everything with plenty of negative anticipatory thoughts.

Mona's husband is also Lebanese and Christian and, similar to Mona, works in a company as a director in charge of one of the departments. Mona described her husband as an "educated, traditional, and conservative man with limited interests," while she described herself as a "liberal and sociable woman with many interests and aspirations." She felt that she wanted more than what he could ever offer her; when they first married, she thought he was more financially well-off than the reality. So Mona blames him for her needing to work in order to support the family, while she thought she would not need to work after her marriage. She felt obliged to work since her husband's income alone was not enough to fulfill the financial needs of the household. She liked having a more active social life while he had "no friends" and did not like going out and interacting with people much. She felt that she was more well-traveled and sophisticated intellectually than he was, thus limiting their common points and topics of conversation. She basically did not feel that he enriched her life or added anything of value to it since they got married.

She admitted getting married because she thought she should do so, given that all her siblings were already married. Although she was not the youngest, she was the only one not yet married and, as a result, experienced pressure from family and friends to avoid the risk of becoming *unmarriageable* as she got older. This is quite common among Lebanese families who see the future of their daughter secured within marriage from a financial, emotional, and social point of view. Marriage, for females, also assures they are not a burden on their family. In the Lebanese culture, if an unwed woman's father is not around anymore, usually her brothers or uncles assume the role of caretaker for her. Consequently, the burden of the adult female child is not restricted to the parents. An unmarried woman cannot live alone; she has to live with a relative. Living alone may ruin her reputation as well as bring shame on the family because the chastity of females who live alone and not under the close supervision of family members is questioned by Arab society.

After her marriage started, Mona realized that she and her husband had many differences in background and personality. She blamed her parents for not warning her about this before she got married as her parents were more familiar with her future husband and his family. Despite the differences between the patient and her husband, Mona expressed to the therapist that she accepted the marriage for the sake of her children and because her husband loved her and was also good to her. She reported that her husband was not very understanding of the stressors and pressures surrounding the conflict between him and their son, which have contributed in part to her depression and anxiety. Moreover, given that divorce was not accepted socially nor within the family, Mona did not consider it as an option for her.

The first time she received treatment for depression was one year earlier. She was prescribed medications, which she stopped using six months later due to her parents insisting that she was okay and did not need treatment. However, the discontinued use of medication resulted in panic attacks and a higher level of depression, which led to her current treatment.

The patient reported feeling ambivalent about her relationship with her parents, frequently relying on them to help her with chores and care for the children and the household but at the same time, resenting that they took her away from her husband and her family, insisting that she and the children live with them. Although her parents did not keep her with them by force, they put a great deal of emotional and psychological pressure on her to make the *right choice* and be away from her family, which according to the parents was the source of her problems, especially her husband. Whenever Mona expressed wanting to return home, her parents blamed her for not making the right decision to help herself and for wanting to stay ill.

Mona indicated in one of the therapy sessions that her parents, especially her father, thought poorly of her husband and often talked to him with condescension. The father blamed the husband for Mona's illness and her feeling weak and unmotivated to fight her anxiety and depression to get better. He believed that Mona's problems started after her marriage, and hence, he drew a causal relationship between her husband and her illness. This conclusion, of course, was underlined by a clear dislike of the husband who did not conform to Mona's parents' wishes and who had many fights with them over living arrangements, work choices, financial security, child rearing, and so on. Mona's father blames her husband for not being more financially secure and requiring Mona to work in order to meet the needs of the family. He also did not like the fact that they bought an apartment in a popular part of the city but not in an area as prestigious as the area the parents lived in. Her father thought that her husband was a poor parent and did not know how to manage his son properly, resulting in misbehaviors of the son and in conflicts between the son and his father.

Based on my professional assessment, Mona felt constantly torn between her parents on one hand and her husband and children on the other. She needed her parents in her weak times since her husband was not understanding of her illness, but she also wanted to focus on her own family, improve her relationship with her husband, and care more for her children by being present with them at home. This ambivalence caused Mona a great deal of anxiety and her incapacity to take any stand made her depressed. As a result, she became helpless and let others, namely her parents, make decisions for her and be in charge of her life.

The Context

Given that it is important to understand Mona's case within its cultural context, various aspects of Arab culture are worth mentioning.

First, individual-family interdependence is predominant in the Arab world. The family is an important source of support (emotional, social, and financial) throughout the lives of its members. Hence, individuals grow up to be psychologically reliant on their families throughout the course of their lives. Male family member's reliance and interdependence differs from that of female family members, whereby female children grow up expecting to be more compliant and supportive with their family of origin and their new family (Dwairy, 2006). Mona's inability to make a decision and differentiate between her needs and those of her family is a reflection of her Arab cultural background that prioritizes individual-family interdependence over individual independence (Dwairy, 2006). Mona's submissiveness and her parents assuming the responsibility of protecting and saving her, given that, in their opinion the husband failed to do so, is another illustration of how individuals in Arab culture are not differentiated from the family and tend to submit to the family's authority and values.

Second, a gender and generational hierarchy exists within the family unit where females and younger members are expected to submit to the authority of males and older members. Mona's reluctance to put limits on her father's intrusion into her marriage can be seen as common in the Arab region, where daughters are expected to submit to the father's authority (Dwairy, 2006). Confronting the father or undermining his authority could have led to the loss of the family's emotional support, which, in turn, would place her at odds with others who follow these traditional practices, both of which she desperately needed at the time and was not ready to give up. The generational hierarchy is also reflected by Mona's reliance on her mother to answer questions addressed to her.

Third, marriage is considered central to the lives of women in the Arab world. Arab women seek marriage because it provides them with what singlehood deprives them of, such as sexual and emotional intimacy, more freedom and independence, financial security, higher social status, and children (Dwairy, 2006). Mona's fear of never getting married, which prompted her to rush into a marital union of which she may have been hesitant about, would not be surprising to Arab readers or others familiar with Arab culture, given the centrality of marriage to women in Lebanon.

Fourth, given that in the Arab culture, marriage is more a union of two families rather than two individuals, it is not uncommon for extended family members to interfere with many aspects of the couple's life, sometimes aggravating or even causing marital problems (Abu-Baker, 2003; Abu-Baker, 2005; Dwairy, 2006). There was a destructive element in

Mona's family in that her mother and father involved themselves in her life in ways that were clearly unwelcomed by Mona and her husband. Moreover, and despite Mona's complaints about her husband, she was not willing to dissolve the marriage, consequently, her father's harsh and judgmental attitude toward her and her family and demands of his daughter's whereabouts contributed significantly to Mona's distress. To add to this distress, Mona's parents did not accept Mona's symptoms of depression and anxiety as these problems are considered a mental illness, which is stigmatized in Arab culture. Seeking mental health services embarrasses and threatens the reputation of affected individuals and their families (Abu-Ras, 2003; Endrawes, O'Brien, & Wilkes, 2007). Families with mentally ill members are at high risk of being stigmatized and discriminated against by society (Kadri, Manoudi, Berrada, & Moussaoui, 2004). For instance, having a mental illness may jeopardize the marital prospects of single women as well as the marriage of Arab wives (Al-Krenawi, Graham, Dean, & Eltaiba, 2004; Al-Krenawi & Graham, 2000: Endrawes et al., 2007).

Fifth, divorce is not approved of in Arab culture because it lowers the status of women and puts their reputation at stake (Dwairy, 2006). Arab wives tend to endure the marriage in silence and prioritize the family, primarily the children, over their personal fulfillment (Abu-Baker, 2005). Indeed, those who endure in silence are respected by society and glorified (Abu-Baker, 2005). Mona's rejection of the idea of divorce reflects her tendency to conform to familial and social norms. Her decision to put up with the marriage for the sake of the children clearly illustrates the primacy of the family over the individual.

Finally, in addition to having to endure marital problems in silence to maintain the family's cohesiveness, the mother's role within the Arab family also entails acting as a buffer when problems arise between the father and the children (Dwairy, 2006). She is expected to maintain harmony within the family unit by reinforcing the authority of the father while, at the same time, maintaining closeness with the children (Dwairy, 2006).

Recently, women's role in the Arab world is expanding beyond that of mother and wife (Goveas & Aslam, 2011; Metcalfe, 2008; Moghadam, 2003). The education and employment of women is becoming increasingly common in the region (Moghadam, 2003). However, there are still cultural, religious, and institutional factors hindering the advancement of Arab women in the professional sphere as well as the social expectation of her role being first and foremost a mother and homemaker (Forster & Al-Marzouqi, 2011; Gallant & Pounder, 2008; Metcalfe, 2008; Whiteoak, Crawford, & Mapstone, 2006). This dichotomy places a great deal of stress on mothers who find themselves in ambivalent positions, torn between their husbands and their children, as exemplified by Mona's case.

_____ **The Treatment**

I saw Mona for a total of three months in weekly sessions followed by two biweekly maintenance sessions following the completion of our sessions. Her mother came with her to the first two sessions, then she accompanied her for the next 6 to 7 weeks but waited in the waiting area. When Mona started feeling better and was able to go back to work, she asked her mother to stop accompanying her to therapy. During the last month as well as for the maintenance sessions, Mona came alone unaccompanied, which was one of the first signs of her achieving a healthy level of independence from her family.

In the therapy process, I often involve other key individuals that live with my patients to get a more accurate and complete picture of my patients' symptoms. In Mona's case, when we started, I asked her if her husband could come to one of our sessions so I could meet him and hear his point of view about his relationship with his wife. Mona was open to this suggestion. They came together to the sixth session. Her husband seemed like a very hurt man, who was upset at the level of interference with their marriage by his in-laws. He reported the constant presence of his in-laws in their house and in their lives. He said that her mother always called Mona on the phone to check on her. If Mona went out, it was with her mother, and when Mona had to choose between an outing with her mother and one with her husband, she often chose the former. He admitted that sometimes they were a support for Mona and his family, but more often than not, they imposed themselves and did not leave room for his relationship with Mona. The husband spoke about these matters in front of Mona who agreed with him and seemed to understand his perception of things and how he felt around her family. They both decided to make more time for each other and for her to start putting limits on her parents by saying no to them when she felt like it.

A few weeks later we had another joint session where Mona and her husband also discussed his relationship with their son and the tension and lack of communication between them, which was a major stressor to Mona. I took the session as an opportunity to present some psychoeducational information regarding parenting skills and the experiences of adolescents. This discussion seemed to help both the patient and her husband to gain some insight into a teenager's world and seemed to make it easier for the husband to understand his son and be more willing to make an effort to improve their relationship. In later sessions, Mona stated that her son and husband fought less, that her husband let the son express his opinion more, and that her husband was willing to listen to the son more. He was also trying to find an activity that they could do together to help with their bonding process. She also changed her attitude towards both and did not play the mediator or act as the son's advocate anymore. She aligned herself with her husband and agreed on certain parenting rules, which they both shared with the son and to which he had to abide by. In return, they let him have his outings with his friends within limits and as long as he held his part of the bargain by focusing on his school work.

One of the main treatment goals mutually agreed upon at the outset of therapy involved helping Mona separate from her parents to a certain degree so that some of her stress related to marital discord could be alleviated. As Mona started to separating from her parents, working on her marriage, and getting closer to her husband, her father fought back, and her mother started coming to the sessions, bringing with her messages from the father to the therapist. Her mother spoke of the inability of Mona to care for the family, blamed her husband's lack of support for her daughter's mental problems, and the fact that Mona was still under a considerable amount of pressure and stress. During the sessions, Mona and I talked about her being a mature, highly achieved, independent adult and not a child anymore depending on her parents. Mona's mother was able to see that and agreed to act in accordance with this maturity and independence. I coached her about facing her parents and expressing her needs and the changes which she thought were important to them. Mona asked for a joint session with her mother in order to tell her these issues with the presence and support of the therapist. During the joint session, Mona was able to tell her mother that she and her father were a major source of stress for her. Mona also requested that her parents stay away from her home because she wanted to stay married and care for her family. She talked in a calm and self-assured way, as a woman who knew what she wanted and what was best for her. She emphasized her appreciation for her parents' help, her love for them, and her wish to have them in her life on her terms. During the session, I supported her statements while stressing that both parents' wish was to have her happy and that a balance between her nuclear family and her parents would make her achieve that.

After this session, Mona permanently moved back home with her family. Prior to that session, she had already gone back to work part-time. One day after work she decided to go back to her own house and not her parents. She called her parents and told them that as a trial period, she was going to stay at her own house. However, the trial continued, she visited her parents occasionally, and moved her things back to her own home. When she told me of her permanent decision to stay in her house, I celebrated her decision and encouraged her to pursue her efforts by working on her own family issues and putting limits to her parents in an assertive and gentle way.

After moving out from her parents' house, Mona's father increased his phone calls and visits to their house and had many fights with her husband. At some point, he wanted to bring Mona back to their house almost by force. Mona refused and, for the first time, stood between her father and husband and said "no" to her father in his face. She also put limits to her mother, refused to see her daily, and decreased her phone contact despite her parents putting more pressure on her to go back to them. In the sessions, we talked about her feeling guilty towards her parents and sometimes doubting her decision to be with her husband and children. I always reframed her thoughts into the context of her being a mature adult woman knowing what she wanted and making her own choices, needing to make her needs a priority in order for her to feel better. In return, she took initiative to see her parents when she wanted to, invited them to her home, cooked dinner (something she had not done in months), and also spent quality time with her mother at her leisure.

As we went through the therapy process, Mona realized the role her parents played in her marriage problems and her mental problems and decided to put an end to that. We discussed the importance of focusing on one's own family, the nuclear family, which becomes the priority over the extended family of origin. However, this is done without undermining the presence of the family of origin, which usually plays a supportive role to the nuclear family, enriching it on an emotional, social, and sometimes financial level but never hinders the blossoming of the nuclear family, which is what her parents were doing. As Mona realized what her parents were doing, she strived to achieve a better balance in her relationship with her parents and her husband.

Her functioning was an ultimate proof of her demands. She went to her work regularly and she cared for the household, her children, their needs, and her husband's needs. She also spent more time with her children and husband, talking and listening to their concerns and about their lives. Upon my request, she managed to have weekly dates with her husband where they went out as a couple and enjoyed themselves by spending some quality time together away from the daily sources of stress.

After a while, Mona's parents accepted her changes, reluctantly at first, then willingly as they saw her improvement and her being happier in her life. They respected her wishes of needing a little bit more privacy and boundaries in her relationship with them. They distanced themselves somewhat and saw Mona and her family only when she asked for it or if she invited them over.

Mona's increase in self-esteem and positive self-perception worked like magic on her anxiety symptoms. Finally she felt in control of her life and her wishes, and her marriage and family life went in the direction she hoped for. The changes Mona accomplished also resulted in changes in her husband's personality and behavior. He was communicative and more supportive towards Mona and their son. He was also more willing to go along with Mona's wishes of outings and to have a better social life. Mona's husband came to the realization that by Mona being happier and more satisfied with her life and her relationships, he and the children were also happier.

Upon termination, Mona reported feeling much better, being almost anxiety free, and living her life the way she wanted. She realized that there was a continuous effort which needed to be done with her husband, children, and parents; however, she felt that she had the motivation and the energy to undertake it.

Evaluation of the Treatment

The changes Mona displayed and her reports of feeling better were a clear indication of the success of the treatment. She had the resources needed within herself to apply all the suggestions made in therapy and to take the steps necessary to make such drastic changes in her life. From a family systems' perspective, Mona could be seen as the identified patient within her nuclear family whereby she reflected the husband-son conflict. Once she got sick, the system revolved around her illness and the issues later on were talked about and resolved. All this, however, was encompassed in a larger family system of Mona's family of origin, with their own set of problematic issues. Once focused on Mona's problems, theirs became secondary. Therefore, as a result of the therapy the family system around her also had to change. Despite the initial resistance of her parents, they realized that her changes were lasting and Mona was consistent with her decisions. In my opinion, Mona having a female therapist, who normalized her needs for independence, modified her expectations from being a helpless female, and encouraged her to be more assertive, was quite helpful. So, I could be seen as a role model for her. My consistent attempts at empowering her from the outset of therapy gave me instant credibility as a therapist, despite the fact that I looked a little younger than her. However, my position of therapist and academician overcame the age issue and gave me credibility to her, her husband, and her parents.

Empowerment to Mona developed in the sessions by my constantly reminding her that she had her own voice and that she needed to listen to it. Although her voice was initially covered by her parents', husband's, and even children's, she was able to later on discern hers from theirs and give it more attention. For the first time in her life, she was given the opportunity to ask herself what she wanted, answer it, and more importantly, to act upon it. Empowerment also came from focusing on her achievements and successes, and having them as a constant reminder. A crucial aspect of the treatment was to have her seek independence from her parents without complete alienation and disengagement from them. Finding this balance for her and to make it agreeable to them was quite a challenge. Therapy helped Mona find a way to bridge these two aspects in her life once she saw them as complementary to each other and not as mutually exclusive.

Being Lebanese and having lived in Lebanon for most of my life, I am aware of the way girls and women are socialized in Lebanese culture based on their gender. I viewed Mona as a typical case of an Arab woman struggling between her need for independence and her fear of losing familial support and understood her depression as a normal reaction in a culture that focuses on interpersonal fulfillment against self-fulfillment. A Western or Western-trained therapist who was not familiar with the Arab culture may have misunderstood her and pathologized her dependency and reliance on her family. Being with a Lebanese therapist who also lived in the West and was fluent in English helped Mona express herself in any way she wanted. Thus, although most of the sessions were conducted in Lebanese Arabic, Mona sometimes spoke in English, especially when she had difficulty finding the Arabic equivalent of certain words or expressions, such as *depression* or *anxiety*. Such words in Arabic are usually found in the more formal Arabic version, while the colloquial dialect uses the English words.

This case illustrates the role of the family in the Arab culture, and though often it is a great source of support, it can also be a source of sorrow. Women's education and recruitment into the labor force changed their status and challenged Middle Eastern patriarchy (Moghadam, 1998). The importance of the extended family unit decreased giving way to the nuclear family unit. The Arab family is still central to the lives of individuals in the Middle East yet within the limits of the nuclear family (Moghadam, 2003). This could be a sign of change of the Lebanese family and its focus. It could mean that the priority nowadays is put on the nuclear family ties and demands and less on the family of origin. With Lebanon becoming more industrialized, women participating more frequently in the work force, separation of families due to travel and relocation, and the fast pace of modern life and its daily stressors, a new social structure built on the nuclear family rather than the extended one may have been created.

This trend, therefore, leads to parents, children, and other family members having a different type of relationship: Parents need to learn to give more freedom to their adult children while guiding them. At the same time, adult children need to be able to assert their individual rights and those of their nuclear family members without being in severe conflict with the family and community at large. This, of course, does not mean an emotional distancing from the family of origin. To most Lebanese, the larger family is the main source of emotional, psychological, and social support. The key is to be able to find this fine balance between the nuclear family's needs to grow and mature in a healthy way and the allegiance to the family of origin.

References

Abu-Baker, K. (2003). Marital problems among Arab families: Between cultural and family therapy interventions. *Arab Studies Quarterly, 25*(4), 53–74.

Abu-Baker, K. (2005). The impact of social values on the psychology of gender among Arab couples: A view from psychotherapy. *Israel Journal of Psychiatry & Related Sciences, 42*(2), 106–115.

Abu-Ras, W. (2003). Barriers to services for Arab immigrant battered women in a Detroit suburb. *Journal of Social Work Research and Evaluation, 4*(1), 49–65.

Al-Krenawi, A., & Graham, J. R. (2000). Culturally-sensitive social work practice with Arab clients in mental health settings. *Health and Social Work, 25*(1), 9–22.

Al-Krenawi, A., Graham, J. R., Dean, Y. Z., & Eltaiba, N. (2004). Cross-national study of attitudes towards seeking professional help: Jordan, United Arab Emirates (UAE) and Arabs in Israel. *International Journal of Social Psychiatry, 50,* 102–114.

American Psychological Association. (2002). *American Psychological Association ethical principles of psychologists and code of conduct.* Retrieved from http://www.apa.org/ethics/code/index.aspx

Beck, J. S. (1995). *Cognitive therapy: Basics and beyond.* New York, NY: Guilford

Dwairy, M. (2006). *Counseling and psychotherapy with Arabs and Muslims.* New York, NY: Teachers College.

Endrawes, G., O'Brien, L., & Wilkes, L. (2007). Mental illness and Egyptian families. *International Journal of Mental Health Nursing, 16,* 178–187.

Forster, N., & Al-Marzouqi, A. (2011). An Exploratory study of the underrepresentation of Emirate women in the United Arab Emirates' information technology sector. *Equality, Diversity and Inclusion: An International Journal, 30*(7), 544–562.

Gallant, M., & Pounder, J. S. (2008). The employment of female nationals in the United Arab Emirates (UAE): An analysis of opportunities and barriers. *Education, business and society: Contemporary middle eastern issues, 1*(1), 26–33.

Goveas, S., & Aslam, N. (2011). A role and contributions of women in the Sultanate of Oman. *International Journal of Business and Management, 6*(3), 232–239.

Harb, C., & Smith, P. B. (2008). Self-construals across cultures: Beyond independence–interdependence. *Journal of Cross-Cultural Psychology, 39,* 178–197.

Kadri, N., Manoudi, F., Berrada, S., & Moussaoui, D. (2004). Stigma impact on Moroccan families of patients with schizophrenia. *Canadian Journal of Psychiatry, 49*(9), 625–629.

Metcalfe, B. D. (2008). Women, management and globalization in the Middle East. *Journal of Business Ethics, 83*(1), 85–100.

Moghadam, V. M. (1998). *Women, work and economic reform in the Middle East and North Africa.* Boulder, CO: Lynne Rienner.

Moghadam, V. M. (2003). *Modernizing women: Gender and social change in the Middle East.* Boulder, CO: Lynne Rienner.

Poulin, J. (2009). *Strength-based generalist practice: A collaborative approach.* Belmont, CA: Marcus Boggs.

Rasheed, J. M., Rasheed, M. N., & Marley, J. (2011). *Family therapy: Models and techniques.* Thousand Oaks, CA: Sage.

Teyber, E. (2006). *Interpersonal process in psychotherapy: An integrative model* (5th ed.). Belmont, CA: Thomson Brooks/Cole.

Whiteoak, J. W., Crawford, N. G., & Mapstone, R. H. (2006). Impact of gender and generational differences in work values and attitudes in an Arab culture. *Thunderbird International Business Review, 48*(1), 77–91.

World Health Organization. (2005). *The mental health atlas-2005.* Geneva, Switzerland: Author.

6

College Counseling in China

A Case Study

Changming Duan
Xiaoming Jia
Yujia Lei

Introduction

Counseling, defined as a helping professional practice, started in China just a few decades ago and has been developing exponentially. Nowadays, there are counseling services provided on almost all college and university campuses for students, faculty, and staff (An, Jia, & Yin, 2011). Additionally, various training programs have mushroomed, ranging from on-the-job training, short-term, and periodical courses, to advanced degree programs (MA and PhD) in recent years.

It is important to note that due to the increasing interconnectedness among different countries and nations in today's world, and due to the fact that counseling as a profession and a scientific discipline is well-established in the Western part of the world with a large literature, the development of counseling in China has been heavily influenced by the Western theories and practices (Hou & Zhang, 2007). Such Western influence no doubt helped jump-start the profession in China, but it is imperative not to overlook the fact that the cultural context of China is very different than that in the West, which dictates how counseling is and should be conducted to be effective. Thus, regardless of how much Western influence entered

China, effective practice of counseling shows its uniqueness as a product of the culture. It is not to say, however, that features of counseling in the Western cultures are not present in Chinese counseling. What deserves our research attention and understanding is how the integration between the established counseling literature from the West and Chinese counselors' cultural knowledge about helping relationships in China and Chinese clients' experiences plays out in the counseling process and outcome. The theorists and researchers in the West can learn from how their colleagues in international communities shape counseling practice into a culturally relevant phenomenon for their communities. This knowledge in turn helps with the renewal of counseling theories in the West.

In this chapter, we present a case study of a counseling relationship between a college student client and a counseling center staff counselor and the supervisory relationship between the counselor and a much experienced clinician, a member of the first generation of formally trained professional counseling psychologists. We present the case in a way that provides our readers a glimpse of the counseling process in China and allows them to see some similarities and differences between Chinese and Western counseling and supervision practices as well as some examples of how culture plays an important role in client experiences.

Introduction of the Authors

The first author, Changming Duan, was born and grew up in China. She earned her bachelor's degree from Hefei Polytechnical University in China and graduate degrees from institutions in North America, including her PhD in counseling and social psychology from the University of Maryland at College Park. She is currently an associate professor of counseling psychology at the University of Kansas. Her professional interests include studying counseling processes and outcomes in cultural contexts and understanding counseling practices in her country of origin, China.

The second author, Xiaoming Jia, is the clinical supervisor for the case in this study. She received one bachelor's degree in physics from Beijing Institute of Technology and one in education from Beijing University. For her generation, there were no degree programs in counseling or counseling related fields in China. Xiaoming Jia received systematic training in counseling with an emphasis on person-centered approach and in psychoanalytical theories and practice through various training programs. As a senior visiting scholar, she worked with the counseling psychology program at the University of British Columbia from 1998 to 1999. Currently, Xiaoming Jia is a professor of counseling psychology and the director of the Institute of Applied Psychology on a college campus (name is not presented to protect client identity). She has been engaged in teaching, clinical practice, supervision, and research in counseling psychology for over 20 years. Her research areas include understanding and applying psychoanalysis theories in psychotherapy, psychoanalysis-existential approaches in group counseling, processes and outcomes of college counseling, and bereavement counseling.

Changming Duan knew of Professor Jia's name for a long time due to her high reputation in the field of counseling in China. Professor Jia was a member of the first 2-year-long doctoral level class that received systematic training in counseling, with an emphasis on person-centered approach, cosponsored by Beijing Normal University and the Chinese University in Hong Kong in the1990s. The members of that class have become the leaders in the counseling field, especially in establishing counseling centers on college campuses, developing postgraduate training programs in counseling, and serving as supervisors for clinical trainings throughout China.

When invited by the first author to coauthor this case study, Professor Jia recommended using a case she had supervised. She felt that the case provided a glimpse of counseling processes at college campuses in China both in the types of clients and client concerns and how counselors conduct counseling. This case was deemed as a good illustration because it lasted for 18 sessions (which allows client changes to be observed), the counselor felt challenged while working with the client, the counselor-client working alliance developed gradually, and the client openly showed that he really valued the therapeutic relationship.

The third author, Yujia Lei, was the counselor for the client in this case study. She is a 26-year-old female Chinese native. She received her BA degree in social work and MA degree in counseling psychology from a university in a major city in China (again the name is not presented for protection of client identity). She was an outstanding student in the university, ranking number one in her undergraduate class and very top in her MA program. Thus, she was offered the job to be a staff counselor at the counseling center of the university upon graduation from the MA program (there is a lot of prestige associated with such a job offering), where she saw the client in this study. The termination of the case occurred (the client chose not to transfer to another counselor) when she left the counseling center and enrolled in a PhD program in counseling psychology in the United States.

She received training in various Western counseling theories and techniques during her study in the MA program, which required 36 credit hours of course work, 100 hours of practicum, and completion of a master thesis. In addition, she also received a two-year-long periodic training in psychoanalysis by an American-Chinese training group in China. This training experience included intensive face-to-face training (six days long each time and two times per year) for lectures, supervision, self-analysis, and group discussion. Trainees also participated in ongoing group supervision twice per month for the two-year training period. During group supervision, trainees brought their cases, self-reflection notes, or any questions they had for class discussion and supervision.

As the result of training and her personal experiences, Yujia Lei describes her therapeutic approach as primarily rooted in person-centered theory/ humanistic philosophy with some tenets of psychoanalytic and psychodynamic ways of thinking. She perceives her role as a counselor to be "a traveling companion for her clients on the journey of life." In traveling with clients, she hopes to share clients' pain and provide all the necessary facilitative conditions (Rogers, 1957) in a here-and-now fashion for clients' growth and independence. She has strong faith in the potential and resilience of clients to grow, change, and actualize themselves and believes that exhibiting this faith through the counseling relationship is essential to client growth. Practically, she reports that she often uses psychoanalytic and psychodynamic theories in conceptualizing the sources of her clients' concerns but does not rely on using psychodynamic interventional methods. She sees that an integration of psychodynamic and humanistic theories allows her to try as best as possible to enter the world of clients, acknowledging both weaknesses and strengths of their personalities and ways of coping. In other words, she is interested in understanding the intricacies of what blocks her clients' development yet focuses her attention in sessions on creating an environment of genuineness and authenticity.

The Case

The first author initiated this case study to obtain an in-depth understanding of one counseling relationship at a college counseling center in China. It should be noted that the first author was not involved in any clinical role with this case, and this case study was conducted eight months after the counseling process was terminated. The objectives of the case study include, through an intensive examination of one case, acquiring detailed knowledge about how counseling and supervision are conducted in the setting, how a Chinese counselor who has been trained with Western theories and methods approaches a Chinese client (including conceptualizing client concerns and delivering clinical interventions), how a supervisor operates to contribute to counselor growth and therapeutic outcome, how clients respond to counseling, a process largely perceived as a relatively new phenomenon (often with stigma), and how the therapeutic relationship is viewed by the client and counselor.

Procedure

The process of the counseling was not controlled or manipulated. In fact, the observational data were collected based on retrospective recollections, written case records, session recordings, and supervision notes provided by the counselor and the supervisor. Based on the information provided by these records, the first author conducted interviews with the counselor and the supervisor with a series of questions including the following: What was the counselor's mind set when approaching the case? What was the working conceptualization of the client concerns? What were the ongoing treatment plans and goals, and what theories drove these goals? What were some of the markers of therapeutic outcomes (positive or negative)? What process variables, techniques, or skills likely contributed to positive outcomes? What process variables, techniques, or skills likely contributed to negative outcomes? What are some hypotheses (in terms of the relationship between counseling process and outcome) that could be derived from this experience that are worth future research?

The writing process of the chapter involved Dr. Duan's drafting of what were discussed among the three authors and Professor Jia and Ms. Lei's repetitive review and editing. Many mini follow-up interviews and short discussions occurred during the writing process to gain new knowledge and clarifications. The verbal communication among the authors was primarily in Chinese, mixed with English words and terms.

The Client

The client was a 21-year-old Chinese male college sophomore in a comprehensive university of technology in a major city in China. This university, although not considered as in the Tier I level of universities in China, is a quite prestigious institution that requires high scores from the national entrance examination for admission. The client entered the university as a very top scorer and was awarded the highest level of merit-based scholarship (only the very top few could receive it). He majored in applied physics, which is an extremely competitive major. Students could only be admitted to this major after they proved themselves by earning high marks in their first two years of major studies in sciences. Only the very top few could be admitted each year.

The client presented himself to counseling because of "emotional instability, lack of motivation, and poor self-control" in his own words. He reported that he had not been getting out of bed for about a month and had not been attending classes. There was no report by the client himself and no indication as gleaned by the initial intake interview about any other medical conditions that the client was experiencing.

The client was notably depressed when he entered counseling. He had not shaved for some time and was very thin. He did not make eye contact often when talking to the counselor. He used sophisticated words and complicated sentences, sometimes scientific terms in physics, when talking to the counselor. This presentation seemed to be an attempt to show off his intelligence. He apparently had some knowledge about the counseling process because he was once a member of the student psychological association on campus. He made his knowledge about counseling known by using counseling jargon such as saying that he needed to devote time to long-term counseling to "completely understand myself" and "solve my own problems."

Contextual Conditions

There are many cultural conditions that need to be considered in understanding Chinese clients and their concerns. Among them, we think the following three are particularly relevant to this client's experiences. One of them is that entering a prestigious college is extremely highly regarded and desired but very difficult in China. Differential statuses and levels of prestige of colleges are clearly seen and presented in the society, and entering a highly prestigious one is viewed not only as an indication of the student's great success but also a glory on the face of the whole family. Many parents dream of this high status for their child and are willing to sacrifice anything and everything to support the child's effort. Due to the single-child policy (each couple is allowed to have only one child for the sake of population control) that was strictly enforced during the 1980s and 1990s, many youngsters born in those years were the single child in the family and had to shoulder the heavy responsibility of realizing their parents' dream single-handedly. Moreover, the entrance to college is largely determined by applicants' test scores in the once-a-year national entrance examination. Thus, the pressure to do well on this examination is extremely high and only the most accomplished can enter top or prestigious colleges.

Another condition worth noting is that China has experienced a large and rapid growth economically in recent years, and as a by-product, the economic status of individuals has become more of a salient issue for individuals (Wu & Chen, 2010). This is due to a number of reasons including that the Chinese economic policies in recent years have allowed some people to become richer than others. For a society that has a strong collectivistic tradition and need to maintain sameness and harmony, such status differences create psychological stress and adjustment difficulties for many people, especially those who feel left behind by the economic growth (Yang, 1998). Often times being rich is viewed as being successful and superior, and being poor is viewed as being incapable or a loser.

The third condition is related to the social perception of counseling. In China, counseling on college campuses has been promoted by the government and various educational organizations. On one hand, the climate for counseling and seeking help has been created, but on the other, stigma associated with seeking counseling is still high, and most individuals who experience psychological concerns and difficulties do not seek help (Jiang, Xia, & Duan, 2011). Those who do seek help often expect the counselor to provide solutions to their problems and want to terminate the counseling process as quickly as possible (Qian, Smith, Chen, & Xia, 2002).

The Client in Context

These contextual conditions played a significant role in the client's experiences. The client graduated from one of the most prestigious high schools in the city, where students were selected (based on test scores) from all other high schools in the city, and therefore appeared to be an exceptionally intelligent student. Unfortunately, he did not do as well as he could on the National Physics Olympia Competition or the college entrance examination during his graduating year from the high school. His score, although very high, did not get him in either of the two Tier I universities in China, and he ended up attending a university that was not prestigious enough in his mind. While obtaining good grades and performing at superior levels, he felt very disappointed about the teaching and educational system of his current university—feeling it was not good or challenging enough to do any good for him or other students. Thus, he said he would apply for a PhD program in the United States at one point, not for himself but for "the well-being of the next generation in China" and for "providing good education for young people." Although he eventually revealed that he would not pursue the United States doctorate, he maintained that he wanted to change the current educational system in China.

In terms of his family background, the client reported that his parents were not rich and had little extra money to support his various efforts for self-advancement such as taking GRE preparation classes. Because of the family's relative poverty, he had to use some of his scholarship money to cover his grandma's medical expenses. He seemed to feel embarrassed by what his parents did for living (manual laborers), so he used job titles that reflected some truth but were clearly misleading toward higher social status than the fact to describe his parents' positions on the intake form. The client also reported that his family lived in a suburb of the city, where the life style was "no comparison with the urban life (urban life is much more desirable than suburban life in China)." To some degree, the client seemed to resent the fact that he was reared in a suburb rather than in the city.

Counselor Conceptualization of Client Concerns

Consistent with the humanistic philosophy, the counselor saw the client as needing growth, self-awareness, and stronger ego strength. Adhering to the Chinese value of well-being as functional improvement (rather than fixing or correcting problems), she did not see the need to diagnose him in terms of pathology. The counselor viewed him as being stuck due to many external and internal factors in the course of normal growth and needing assistance to unstick himself to move forward in his development. In other words, the counselor was more in tune to the client's growth and developmental needs than to his perceived problems. The counselor saw her role as a facilitator and collaborator in client growth and to help the client understand himself in a broad social and cultural context.

The counselor was aware that the client felt superior for being extremely intelligent and on the very top of his age group in academic performance, but at the same time, he felt inferior as he failed to earn a top place in the physics Olympic competition in high school and failed to get admission to the very top university in China. The root of his inferiority may be related to his experience of family low social and economic status, parents' high expectations on his academic performance, and the way in which his failure was viewed by the society. The counselor felt that it was largely his social and cultural context that contributed to his level of difficulty in life, although his experience also reflected his weak ego strength. His weak ego strength could be perceived both as a cause for some of his feelings and experiences and a symptom resulting from his interactions with people. The counselor believed that such an understanding of his internal struggle from a dynamic point of view helped her understand the client and empathize with him accurately. The counselor also saw that empathy was what the client needed the most because he, in his position, got little if any empathy or sympathy from others (his intelligence and academic success appeared to have put him above the majority of people in his age group). Empathy and unconditional support, coupled with insights about contextual influences, would facilitate his growth out of the inferiority.

It was truly remarkable in most people's eyes that the client was able to attend the high school that gathered the most elite and promising students. Most of the attending students had exceptionally high IQs and highly respected family backgrounds (i.e., with a high level of education and high income). Attending the school, however, was not without drawback for the client. He reported that besides one excursion sponsored by his mother's company, he had to stay at home during holidays and breaks, whereas most of his classmates went abroad or ventured in other costly activities. This experience probably contributed to his sense of inferiority. Without strong ego strength, the client developed the tendency, often desperately, to seek affirmation of his self-worth and self-value from how others perceived him. He showed signs of intense fear of being looked down upon by others. The client described himself as an *upstart* (someone who became elite without the family-provided foundations that were typically associated with success in China) but was trapped in a cycle of being *upstart-poor-upstart-poor*. He said that he felt like an upstart when competing with less-intelligent peers but felt poor when competing with more-intelligent others, feeling superior and inferior accordingly. Both in his external and internal worlds, he experienced ups and downs in his performances and in his feelings about himself. He admitted that he looked down upon ordinary students but was scared to compete with extraordinary people.

The counselor also saw reflection of the client's weak ego in the interpersonal difficulties that he presented in sessions. He had few friends and felt close to no one on campus. He said he wanted to be helpful to others but felt unappreciated when he offered help. For instance, he said he always wanted to help his classmates expand their knowledge and ideas because "they need to know more," but when he made efforts to teach them, they turned their ears away and even avoided him, which made him angry. From his description, the counselor saw his difficulty in viewing himself as being equal to or at the same level with his peers, which reflected his fear and insecurity in interpersonal relationships. The client showed no awareness of his own need to maintain his sense of superiority and never examined how he may have come across as arrogant when interacting with peers.

The same interpersonal pattern also appeared in his romantic relationships. The client defined himself as both an actor and a director in intimate relationships. In dating females, he reported that once he finished "calculation" of a girl, he lost interest in her. The client's relationship pattern showed that he needed to feel in control and on top of interpersonal relationships, another indication of his insecurity. The client was not aware that his need to be in control and on top created an unequal position for the other party and kept others away from him.

The counselor reported that throughout the counseling process, she found herself seeking answers about what blocked the client's development of a healthy ego and what he needed in order to grow. She felt the family, social, and cultural conditions were largely responsible for the lack of freedom the client experienced in his development. He wanted to be successful and be a good student, which was defined by the culture he was in with objective criteria such as obedience to parents and teachers and superior academic performance (e.g., extraordinary test scores and grade rankings). In such an academic achievement-oriented culture, many students have to pay a high price to become successful, focusing only on numerous academic tests and competitions and not having opportunities to develop interpersonal and social skills. As a result, many achieve high IQ and become book worms but experience low emotional quotient or EQ, not knowing how to deal with failures or interpersonal relationships. This client appeared to be an example of such a cultural product; he did all he was expected to do academically but could not help feeling depressed and insecure and had a lack of direction in life.

The Context

At college counseling centers in China, counseling is usually provided by staff counselors who need to have a minimum of a master's degree to qualify for these professional positions or by practicum students from the MA or PhD programs in counseling psychology. There usually is a senior faculty member responsible for supervising all staff counselors and practicum students. Enrolled students on campus may receive counseling service for free for eight sessions and pay a nominal fee for additional sessions.

Standard counseling sessions are conducted once a week and for 50 minutes per session. Audio and video recording is usually required for junior staff counselors and practicum students for the purpose of receiving supervision from the senior faculty member of the center. Supervision is usually provided in either an individual or group format. For this case study, the supervisor, the second author of this chapter, is a professor in the academic MA training program in counseling psychology for the university and the director of the counseling center. She is one of the few dozens of master supervisors in China who are licensed by the Division of Counseling and Clinical Psychology of Chinese Association of Psychology. She provided supervision in a group format for this case.

The Treatment

To help the client develop a sense of security and feel free to grow, the counselor focused the treatment on establishing a personal connection with him, which was an unfamiliar experience for the client. Strategically, she focused on being attentive, listening, and conveying warmth and unconditional positive regards. She never expressed judgment or criticized him even when he was critical of himself, the counselor, or others. Instead, she showed understanding, empathic emotions, and validation to all his emotions and thoughts regardless of how he experienced and expressed them. Although he displayed narcissism and arrogance sometimes, the counselor genuinely appreciated him and his strengths—he was hard working, academically talented, self-reflective, and over time, became gradually more open. She also felt empathic about his struggles, which she saw largely as stemming from the educational system and social and cultural environment. The counselor reflected that her focus on connection building was present for all 18 sessions, including all three stages of counseling as identified by Hill (2009), namely the beginning stage, working stage, and termination stage. With supervision, the counselor felt that her effort in establishing an effective therapeutic relationship with the client became more successful as the counseling process unfolded.

In group supervision, through the observation of both verbal and nonverbal exchanges between the client and the counselor, the supervisor helped the counselor further understand the core issues that the client was struggling with and both the internal and external processes he experienced. Based on the content of the client's reports, his nonstop talking pattern during the earlier stage of counseling, the counselor's difficulty in feeling close to the client, and the way the two communicated nonverbally (e.g., in one session, the client leaned forward while talking and the counselor sat back with a cup in hand), the supervisor hypothesized that the client's core issues were (1) self-centeredness and (2) identity crisis. In collaboration with the counselor, the supervisor presented a conceptualization of the client as illustrated by Figure 6.1.

As shown by the figure, the client's struggles resulted from and reflected in two groups of factors: intra- and interpersonal factors and counseling-process-related factors. The intrapersonal factors included feeling inferior due to family background (and possibly lack of close relationships with parents), lack of meaningful interpersonal relationships, superior yet not good enough academic performance, conflictual feelings about seeking help (wanting help but needing to feel superior), and past experiences of injuries from interpersonal interactions in various areas of life. These internal processes were stressors for the client because they reflected his failures in meeting the perceived social and cultural expectations. Subsequently, the following behavioral patterns of the client were observed in counseling. He came to counseling only because he could not pull himself out of obviously wrong and unacceptable behavior (e.g., staying in bed and not going to classes). In counseling, he showed off his intellectual ability by using sophisticated statements, big words, and psychological jargon to tell well-articulated stories, showed the counselor his competitiveness, and often changed topics in order to stay in control and avoid going deep into any topic.

The supervisor emphasized the importance of helping the client develop empathy (which would help him be less self-indulgent and see himself in relation to others, e.g., a person with strengths and weaknesses just like

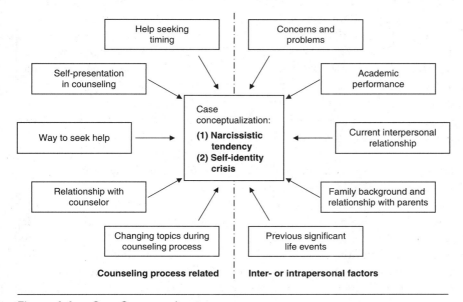

Figure 6.1 Case Conceptualization

everyone else). Both the supervisor and the counselor agreed that the best way to approach this goal was through counselor modeling of empathy. The supervisor helped the counselor see that the client's nonstop talking in early sessions reflected his need to show his intelligence and ability. Such behavior was probably a demonstration that the client felt threatened by the counselor because she was well-known on campus and regarded as highly intelligent with an outstanding academic record. The supervisor suggested that instead of directly interpreting the client experience or directing him to reduce his self-centeredness, using empathy would be most helpful in helping him feel validated, respected, and understood. In other words, leading him toward a positive direction was more effective than pointing out what was wrong with his direction at the time because he was defensive and insecure and would not listen to comments about him being wrong. Consistent with the counselor's person-centered orientation and the client's personal style, the supervisor emphasized the importance of the counselor joining in with the client. Both the supervisor and the counselor agreed that understanding the client's issues of ego strength and unconscious motives would help the counselor better grasp the client's phenomenology and use both cognitive and emotional empathy effectively. The supervisor believed that counselor's empathy and unconditional acceptance would afford the client an opportunity to experience an authentic and genuinely caring relationship, which could provide the client with some corrective experience. Ultimately, they hoped that the client would learn from the counselor and develop empathy toward others in interpersonal relationships.

The counselor continued to focus on empathizing with the client, showing respect to him regardless of how competitive or insecure he behaved in sessions. Gradually, the client was more able to face his own vulnerability. He began to explore his ideas and behaviors in interpersonal relationships. The client disclosed significant difficulty in establishing meaningful relationships with people, especially women. He said he spent most of his time alone in the library and had little interaction with classmates or roommates. In relating to women, potential romantic partners, he relied mainly on online interactions. He referred to the few women he had such relationships with in the past as *only good for calculations*. His relationships with them were reported to be "really short." He did not seem to feel comfortable with lasting relationships, although he indicated that he really wanted to have a steady romantic relationship with a woman.

The client made noticeable functional progress but showed ups and downs in his behavior both in and outside of counseling sessions. He started going to classes after several sessions but periodically would come to counseling poorly groomed and in a bad mood, complaining of difficulty getting himself motivated to get out of bed. The counselor was determined to offer him complete acceptance and respect and strengthen the therapeutic relationship with him by validating his experiences, rather than offering solutions to solve his problems. With help from the supervisor, the counselor was able to empathize with the client from a cultural perspective, helping the client see how his social and cultural contexts had shaped him and his behavior. For example, when the client criticized himself for having poor self-control, the counselor helped the client see his complaint in the cultural context. When children are raised to work for straight "A" grades in school and to make parents proud by achieving academically, self-discipline and self-demand are heavily emphasized in child rearing but self-nurturance is not. Therefore, the client probably had more difficulty with the self-perception than with the fact of being weak in self-control. In Chinese culture, being self-critical is often considered a responsible way to respond to stress. Self-doubt or uncertainty about self-identity can be the outgrowth of stress related to the cultural environment. In addition, even though family dynamics are clearly affected by the environment and each dynamic making up this nested system of influences to the overall person, the counselor perceives greater success in therapy when personal and family conditions are generally avoided. In sessions, the counselor never directly addressed his lack of motivation or low self-esteem, instead she focused on validating and accepting him as a person. This was consistent with the humanistic conceptualization that the client needed assistance in developing and growing and with the Chinese value of an indirect communication style, especially in communicating expectations (Zhang, Li, & Yuan, 2001). The client seemed to respond to such interventions well. He was engaged in and motivated to pursue the counseling process and showed willingness to explore his weaknesses.

During the course of counseling, the counselor also sought supervision in several specific areas. First, the counselor was not sure about how to approach the client's difficulty in talking about his family and his feelings about his family. From the case conceptualization, the client's feelings about his family background were certainly an area of concern and were contributing factors to his feelings of inferiority. It was a particularly sensitive area for discussion, however, due to the cultural expectation that one should protect one's family's face. It is absolutely not acceptable in China for people to feel shameful about their parents. One can't choose one's parents and negating parents equals negating oneself. The supervisor reminded the counselor that an empathic response should include seeing the client's difficulty as rooted in the cultural context, which must be appreciated and respected. This mind-set helped the counselor recognize such dynamics and be patient with the client. She genuinely felt okay that the client did not need to talk about his family until he was ready to initiate it. The counselor later reflected that how she approached this area of concern was not consistent with the psychodynamic point of view that the client needs to be provided with corrective experience while reliving the life experience that had caused difficulty in the past. In this case, it would involve the client talking about how his family being poor had caused him embarrassment or shame when he was younger.

Another question the counselor brought to supervision was her discomfort with the topic of sex. As the client became comfortable in sessions, he disclosed having strong sexual desires for women, which were not fulfilled due to the lack of steady romantic relationships. Talking about sex openly is generally not acceptable and talking about it with a person of opposite sex of similar age is definitely deemed improper in Chinese culture. The counselor reported receiving no training in this area in graduate school. Therefore, she said she "failed to show interest in the topic when the client brought it up for the first time," which probably led to the client's silence about it in subsequent sessions. The supervisor discussed the possibility that the client, with his self-perceived extraordinary talent, needed to maintain the self-image of being pure and perfect. Discussing sex was risky for him because wanting to have sex could be seen as entering the forbidden zone or doing the unspeakable. The supervisor recognized that the fact the client brought up the topic was a significant sign of progress. The counselor's discomfort probably reflected her internal conflict and stress related to her own ability to face this issue, which was somewhat similar to what the client experienced. The supervisor suggested that the counselor admit having difficulty with talking about sex (normalizing the culturally unacceptable behavior) with the client and ask the client if he felt the same way. Again, this was a strategic and indirect (consistent with the cultural value) way of communicating thoughts about a taboo subject. Unfortunately, as the termination was near, the counselor did not get to explore this with the client.

Both the counselor and the supervisor were quite aware of the gender issues while working with the client. In Chinese society, men are often perceived as having higher social power than their female counterparts (Tang, Chua, & O, 2010). This is especially true in an institute of technology where the majority of the student body is male. When a male student sees a female counselor, the power hierarchy can potentially change. In this case, both the counselor (who was a graduate of the institute) and the client had to adjust to their newly acquired power position—with the female being on the top of the power structure. Throughout the counseling process, the supervisor and the counselor watched for transference and countertransference closely and analyzed any signs of those feelings. The counselor recognized that her discomfort with talking about sex was partially due to her self-perceived female social roles (e.g., females should not talk about sex with males) and maybe somewhat due to her lack of adjustment to the new power structure as well. The supervisor helped the counselor see that the client tried to be both the director and the actor (as he reportedly did in his relationships with other women) so he would not feel weak or powerless in their relationship. He brought up various topics to set the agenda for counseling and then left them for the counselor to figure out the issues in those areas to offer him empathy and understanding. In some ways, the client really enjoyed the deepening and enduring therapeutic relationship with the counselor as an actor because he was never able to keep long-term relationships with his previous girlfriends. His attachment to the counselor may have been one of the reasons that he refused to be transferred to another counselor when the counselor had to leave the center. Unfortunately, there was no opportunity to explore that theory after the termination.

Evaluation of the Treatment

Consistent with psychoanalytic-humanistic conceptualization, the counselor and supervisor both evaluated the effectiveness of the treatment in the context of client growth. Throughout the counseling, the client showed the following positive signs of growth:

1. The client consistently attended counseling, even during the time that he had difficulty getting out of bed. The client reported looking forward to the "start of living" on Thursdays (counseling sessions occurred on Thursdays). Even though he showed his competitive nature with counselor who was known to have an outstanding academic record, he was able to overcome feelings of threat and attended 18 counseling sessions without missing appointments.

2. The client changed his verbal communication style as the treatment progressed. During the early sessions, he talked continuously about the evolution of his problems and their logical consequences without emotion. Gradually, he showed some feelings. He acknowledged he had weaknesses, inferiority, and fear, although his expression of those feelings was still indirect. For example, he wrote and shared a poem, "Spring Comes," to describe his emotions and hope for the future.

3. The client gradually developed some level of self-acceptance for his imperfection and uncertainty. His rigidity in thinking and intolerance of was more flexible in his perception of life, seeing there were more choices and paths toward success in life than before.

4. The client showed some willingness to reach out—moving away from a high level of self-focus to some other- and system-focused interest. For instance, during treatment, he talked about his family and interpersonal relationships and made some effort to connect with others through both in-person and online forums and with the society by showing interest in what was going on in the news. Notably, he still talked a lot about his "struggling cycle" that "conquered or defeated him," but he was more willing to shift the focus to his relationship with the outside world.

5. The client clearly gained some courage in sharing and discussing negative life events and his frustration and inability to maintain interpersonal relationships, especially his feelings about and

relationships with women. He feared involvement in intimate relationships but sought it through online means all the time. Through talking about his feelings in sessions, he developed the insight that what he desired was sincere and caring relationships with women. He was able to disclose that he did not help in this desire—that he did not extend this care in his past relationships.

6. The client appeared to handle the termination of the counseling due to the counselor's departure well. In the context of the client's competitive nature, this could be perceived as a reflection of progress. This was the first and only counseling relationship the client ever had, and he took risks to invest in it. The client felt comfortable leaving counseling at the time (instead of seeing another counselor at the center). He verbalized his thoughts in the last counseling session: "Counseling is like a piece of cloth, wiping every corner of my heart, even some invisible parts. What's more, I have the chance to face the reality and my past again, which I was afraid of before. Living through so much reflection is being reborn."

Conclusion

In retrospection, the counselor focused on the challenges she experienced during the course of treatment in earning the client's trust and establishing working alliance. She felt her conceptualization of the client as someone facing challenges in developing a stronger ego and becoming relationship focused (instead of highly self-centered) helped her provide the client with the necessary conditions for change. The psychodynamic appraisals of the client helped her experience and express empathy accurately and offer her support effectively. Showing respect and appreciation along with empathy appeared to be the most important element of the interventions that led to the observed positive outcomes.

Additionally, the counselor recognized that the social and cultural conditions played an important role in the life of this client. Being academically intelligent and achieving highly is extremely highly regarded in China, which led to the client feeling a sense of superiority. However, the limitation in financial resources and low social status of his parents' occupations or living conditions likely created a feeling of inferiority, which has become a salient issue for many people in China in recent years. These polarized and conflicted feelings can contribute to difficulties in defining the self. The experiences of the client in this study exemplified the psychological complex created by these internal conflicts.

Based on her clinical experiences, the counselor provided the following observations for research about and practice with college students who experience psychological health concerns in China:

1. Academically talented and top-ranked students are adored by parents, peers, teachers, and the society. It is not well acknowledged,

however, that the demand for achieving such high status creates high psychological stress for students. As a result, many students internalize the societal demand and impose a high level of self-demand on academic performance, which can be costly in terms of their general psychological development. For example, the client in this case study calculated when it was the best time to go to the cafeteria when the line was shortest so he could save five or ten minutes to study more. He rigidly scheduled his study from 7:00 a.m. to 11:00 p.m. without group study, discussion, breaks, or social activities. Such high intensity in studying is accompanied with high psychological vigilance and intensity and can lead to burn out. Failure to meet the high goal after such intense investment can lead to self-doubt and a sense of inferiority (Costigan, Hua, & Su, 2010).

2. Prevention and intervention at the system or policy levels is needed for psychologically helping Chinese college students. Individual students should not be blamed for pursuing academic excellence at the cost of social life and personal mental health. In fact, high-performing students should be commended for being willing to sacrifice their personal interest and health for adjusting to social and cultural expectations. It is the academic evaluation system and standards that need to be revisited to reduce pressure for students. The client in this case study once said, "We were educated to focus on studying when we were kids. The higher grade you get, the higher IQ you have, and the better student you are. The attitudes were deep-rooted, although I doubted about it. I feel both confident and inferior. In others' eyes, I am good with excellent abilities, but I know I am weak internally." Obviously, psychological support for high achieving students needs to happen at the system level. The education, evaluation, and reward system (e.g., college admission standards) needs to aim at promoting diverse interests and skills in defining good or successful students (such effort may help change social and cultural expectations for students) and educating students about the importance of psychological health. The psychological services are needed to validate students' struggles in meeting various expectations placed on them.

3. The psychological needs of gifted students at college deserve research attention. Gifted students often find themselves in an educational environment that does not provide enough intellectual challenge and stimulation and feel lost in achieving fulfillment of their potentials and dreams. Both preventive support programs (e.g., individualized educational plans) and counseling services may be needed to help these students adjust to and continue to develop their talent in the environment. After all, everyone has the need to fulfill his or her potential and the gifted are no exception.

4. Generally, caution is needed in probing and discussing issues related to the family of origin in counseling Chinese people when there are no obvious glories about the family the client can share. It was

extremely difficult for the client in this case study to talk about his parents. He noticeably felt embarrassed when talking about his parents, which did not appear to be an indication of poor family relationships. He stated he was self-managed and self-educated, avoiding saying anything negative about his family. Complaining about the family violated the principle of *filial piety*, which is perceived as immoral or wrong. Additionally, the client seemed to buy into the societal values about education and wealth. For instance, to prevent a loss of respect for his family, the client found many excuses to rationalize his decision to give up the idea of pursuing a PhD study in the United States (for which he had cited financial difficulties before). Psychological education and philosophical discussion on topics such as the meaning of life or the meaning of self-actualization may be helpful for young people. In traditional Chinese culture, topics focusing on the individual or self are not often discussed. However, with the social changes that have been introduced in China in recent years, certain individualistic values have become more acceptable. Education and advocacy that help individuals make sense of their social environment are necessary in addressing both social issues and issues related to individuals' mental health.

References

An, Q., Jia, X., & Yin, H. (2011). Professional competence and development of college counselor. *Psychological Science, 34* (2), 107–112. (Published in Chinese in China)

Costigan, C. L., Hua, J. M., & Su, T. F. (2010). Living up to expectations: The strengths and challenges experienced by Chinese Canadian Students. *Canadian Journal of School Psychology, 25*(3), 223–245. doi:10.1177/0829573510368941

Hill, C.A. (2009). *Helping skills: Facilitating exploration, insight, and action* (3rd ed.). Washington, DC: American Psychological Association.

Hou, Z. J., & Zhang, N. (2007). Counselling psychology in China. *Applied Psychology: An International Review, 56,* 33–50.

Jiang, G. R., Xia, M., & Duan, C. (2011). *Relationships among attribution of psychological problems, self-efficacy of being a counseling client, perceived social acceptance of help-seeking, and actual help-seeking behavior among Chinese college students.* Manuscript submitted for publication.

Qian, M., Smith, C. W., Chen, Z., & Xia, G. (2002). Psychotherapy in China: A review of its history and contemporary directions. *International Journal of Mental Health, 30,* 49–68.

Rogers, C. R. (1957). The necessary and sufficient conditions of therapeutic personality change. *Journal of Consulting Psychology, 21,* 95–103.

Tang, C., Chua, Z., & O, J. (2010). A gender perspective on Chinese social relationships and behavior. In M. Bond (Ed.), *The Oxford handbook of Chinese psychology (pp. 533–553).* New York, NY: Oxford University Press.

Wu, P., & Chen, G. (2010). Investigation of psychological health condition of undergraduate students in Shanghai universities. *Journal of Shanghai Jiaotong University, 3*(8), 906–909. (Published in Chinese in China)

Yang, K. (1998). Chinese responses to modernization: A psychological analysis. *Asian Journal of Social Psychology, 1*(1), 75–97. doi:10.1111/1467-839X.00006

Zhang, N., Li, Q., & Yuan, Y. (2001). Expectation of folks on psychotherapy and counseling. *Chinese Mental Health Journal, 15*(4), 250–252. (Published in Chinese in China)

7

Counseling a Female Client From Korea

Applying the Han Counseling Model

Lawrence H. Gerstein
Young Soon Kim
TaeSun Kim

This chapter highlights the work of a highly esteemed mental health professional in Korea. The case of a female Korean client is presented. One of the few indigenous models of Korean counseling is introduced and also discussed in relation to the counseling process with the featured client. The effectiveness of this indigenous approach is discussed as well.

Introduction of the Authors

Lawrence (Larry) was raised in a lower middle class neighborhood in Brooklyn, New York. He earned a BBA degree in public administration with a minor in psychology from Bernard Baruch College in New York and in 1974 completed an MA degree in rehabilitation counseling from the University of Georgia. After practicing as a substance abuse counselor and private clinician for many years, Larry returned to the University of Georgia and earned a PhD in counseling and social psychology in 1983.

Larry completed his predoctoral internship at the Counseling Center at Southern Illinois University–Carbondale. In 1983, he became a faculty member in the department of Counseling Psychology and Guidance Services at Ball State University (BSU). Currently, Larry is a George and Frances Ball Distinguished Professor of Psychology-Counseling at BSU and he directs the doctoral program in counseling psychology and the Center for Peace and Conflict Studies. For over 30 years, Larry has consulted worldwide with educators, psychologists, social workers, and counselors. He is the founding co-chair of the American Psychological Association Society of Counseling Psychology International Section and the co-editor of the *Counseling Psychologist-International Forum*. In 2009, Larry co-edited the *International Handbook of Cross-Cultural Counseling: Cultural Assumptions and Practices Worldwide,* and in 2011 he served as a co-editor of *Essentials of Cross-Cultural Counseling.* Larry connected with Young Soon Kim as a result of a recommendation made by his former doctoral student Dr. Seong-in Choi. In 2007, Young Soon invited Larry to conduct a solution-focused workshop in Seoul, Korea, for the Han Counseling Association.

Since conducting the workshop, Young Soon and Larry have collaborated on projects and interacted with each other at professional meetings in Korea and the United States. Although Larry has not directly observed Young Soon in a counseling situation, he recognizes that Young Soon is a highly talented and greatly admired mental health provider, educator, supervisor, and administrator. Through his experience and observation when others are in her presence, Larry has realized Young Soon is extremely empathic, respectful, warm, accepting, curious, creative, genuine, humble, dynamic, and excellent in her ability to generate solutions when presented with challenges. Others respond to Young Soon with admiration, deep respect, and behaviors that convey she is perceived as one of the primary leaders of the mental health profession in Korea.

Young Soon Kim was born in Seoul, Korea, and currently lives in Cheonan, Korea. She majored in psychology at Chung-Ang University where she earned her bachelor's and master's degrees. For her PhD, she studied counseling psychology in the education department at Wonkwang University. Her dissertation focused on the development and effects of a group counseling parenting program based on reality therapy. The program taught attendees effective parenting skills for dealing with their delinquent adolescent offspring.

Young Soon performs individual and group counseling with adolescents and their parents targeting a variety of issues (e.g., internet abuse and addiction, academic concerns, delinquency, interpersonal relationships, career concerns, and so on). She worked as an instructor and counselor at the Masan Loveaid Foundation, a researcher at the Kyung-nam Family Therapy Center, and for the past 17 years as a chief at the Chung-nam

Youth Counseling Center in Cheonan, Korea. She also has taught psychology, group counseling, and family counseling in the undergraduate and graduate programs in the psychology and education departments at Chungnam National University, Kyungnam University, Soonchunhyang University, and Hoseo University. Young Soon served as the chair of the Han Counseling Association from 2006 to 2010.

As a chief at the Chnug-nam Youth Fostering Center, she is a head of counseling and youth policy-related teams. Young Soon is called *Chief* when she is counseling a client since this is her official name at the center. As chief, she is involved in and supervises projects including the 1388 youth hotline. The hotline (telephone number 1388) is a service for individual youth counseling, crisis counseling, harmful environment reporting, and providing information. As chief, Young Soon also manages the Community Youth Safety Net (CYS-Net). This is a network for preventing and intervening in a crisis for youth. Young Soon also networks with related agencies, supervises and educates counselors, and provides counseling to clients. Because of her other tasks, counseling is not Young Soon's main job. She spends about 5 hours per week in counseling-related work including counseling clients and supervising counselors.

Generally, clients are referred to counselors by their teachers, the youth hotline, and by acquaintances. Other counseling professionals or acquaintances refer about one-half of Young Soon's clients. Young Soon believes this is atypical of other Korean counselors. She thinks her expertise may explain how she gets referrals. Young Soon is often asked, "Could you see my friend?" or "I heard you are an expert. May I see you?" Her counselor friend referred the client presented in this chapter to Young Soon. Young Soon also provides counseling to trainees. Many counseling programs she is connected to encourage trainees to attend five sessions of counseling for educational purposes. Since Young Soon's center focuses on youth, the majority of her clients are middle school, high school, and elementary school students, 26%, 17%, and 17%, respectively.

TaeSun Kim is one of Larry's current doctoral advisees. She met Young Soon when they began working on this chapter together. TaeSun Kim was born in Seoul. She earned a BA degree in law from Hanyang University and majored in educational counseling for her master's degree at Seoul National University, a degree she earned in 2003. She worked as a counselor and researcher for four years at the Korea Youth Counseling Institute. This is a government agency for youth in Korea. In 2008, she went to the United States to pursue her doctoral degree in counseling psychology with a cognate in social justice at BSU. TaeSun and Larry are in the process of conducting research in Korea on vocational calling, mental health help-seeking behaviors and attitudes, and the use of nonviolence to resolve conflicts. She assisted in the communication between Dr. Gerstein and Dr. Young Soon Kim on this chapter. More specifically, TaeSun helped with identifying topics discussed in the chapter, interviewed Dr. Kim in Korean, and translated Dr. Kim's interview and responses to emails into English. She also contributed content about the Korean culture and current counseling practices.

The Practitioner

Young Soon has various titles from associations like counseling psychologist (Korean Counseling Psychological Association), certified couple and family counselor, Han counseling supervisor (Han Counselling Association), Korean counseling children and adolescence counseling supervisor (Korea Counseling Association), family counseling supervisor (Korea Association of Family Counseling), first-grade group counseling specialist (Korea Counseling Association), nationally certified counselor for youth (Ministry of Gender Equality & Family), and reality therapy certification instructor (William Glasser Institute).

In her clinical practice, Young Soon observed that persons receiving counseling were surprised by how much they changed. They claimed never experiencing such peace in their lives. Clients also felt they always had struggled and were overwhelmed with pressure to succeed and felt sorry for their circumstances. Further, Young Soon learned from her clients that they were better at managing their lives and taking care of themselves after counseling. Clients also told her their friends and family members noticed the positive effects of counseling from their peaceful faces, their increased smiles, and their more relaxed attitudes. Young Soon discovered her clients were relieved because they felt they were accepted the way they were and they were appreciated despite being imperfect. Young Soon also discovered her clients worked hard to prove their value while realizing they did not need to do anything to be loved. She believes her empathetic understanding and respect displayed toward her clients enabled these changes to occur.

Han Counseling Model

Early in her career, Young Soon relied on Carl Rogers's person-centered and William Glasser's reality therapy approaches. Because she found Rogers's approach insufficient when helping youth implement specific behavioral changes and Glasser's strategies lacking in the depth of empathy she could express to her clients, Young Soon embraced a Korean indigenous counseling approach known as Han Ideology (Kim, 1986). She searched for over ten years for a model that fit the Korean culture and emotions and then discovered and learned the Han counseling model. This model was developed and advanced by Dong Su Yoo. Young Soon helped to introduce this model worldwide and in Korea.

The Han counseling model is based on Korean or Han ideology (Kim, 1986). The uniqueness of the Korean way of thought is reflected in Han ideology, especially in its name *Han*. In Korean, *Han* refers to various meanings including big, one, unlimited, many, a few, certain, same, and middle. As Han encompasses very different meanings such as one and many, being a Han person implies various meanings (Kim, 1982). In fact, Han is thought to be a human being as well as a heaven that embraces the world. A human can reach heaven through a Han spirit. Then, the purpose of life is to be a Han person who reaches a heaven (Yoo, Kim, & Lee, 2008). Initially, the model was called oneness counseling, but recently it changed to Han counseling. Han ideology was identified in three of the oldest scriptures in Korea, Chun-Bu-Kyung, Sam-Il-Sin-Go, and Cham-Jun-Gye-Gyeng (Choi, Dong Hwan, 1991, 1996).

These scriptures came from heaven, explaining the will of heaven and Korean collective unconscious. Dangun, a grandson of heaven, built Gojoseon, the first Korean kingdom in 2333 BC (Korea Tourism Organization, 2011) and he provided these scriptures. These scriptures include a traditional Korean value, Hongik Ingan Ewah Saegae. This refers to promoting a broad benefit for all human beings and rightfully harmonizing the world. In these scriptures, a person embraces heaven, earth, and humans (Yoo, 2002). Specifically, it is written in the Chun-Bu-Kyung scripture how human beings and the universe were generated. The Sam-Il-Sin-Go scripture describes how life is precious and that being a human being is a blessing (Choi, 1991). The Cham-Jun-Gye-Gyeng scripture introduces the belief that there are 366 things to do (e.g., human beings should strive to maintain the pure character given to them by heaven) and that human beings should do these in their lives (Choi, 1996).

The Han ideology, therefore, points out that humans are a part of the universe. It indicates that humans are the most significant beings and integrated in terms of heaven, earth, and the universe. According to the Chun-Bu-Kyung scripture, humans are heaven and they actualize and aggrandize heaven's will. Further, human beings have two aspects, a "small self" and the "large (or the true) self." The large self refers to the entire universe and an optimal realization status. Thus, human beings are born as a small self and they pursue being a large self (Yoo et al., 2008). This is the goal of Han counseling. The model could be called *growth-oriented counseling,* since it posits the personal growth of a client leads to the person addressing his or her own issues. This assumption is derived from the Eastern ideology of person-centered counseling that encourages a person's growth rather than the resolution of a problem (Yoo et al., 2008).

There are five stages of counseling linked with the Han model: preparing for counseling, developing the relationship, evaluating the problem, intervening, and termination. In the preparation stage, the counselor gathers as much information as possible including the client's motivation for counseling, his or her personality characteristics, the potential prognosis, and the presenting problems. Young Soon believes because a client may state different information depending on levels of intimacy and rapport, the counselor needs to consider these influences. In the developing relationship stage, the counselor builds rapport with the client and sets goals for counseling. In the evaluation stage, Young Soon has discovered it is important to include the client and counselor perspective related to evaluating the problems. During the intervention stage, the counselor addresses the client's presenting problem as relayed by the client and not the counselor. Then, when the client is ready to listen to another perspective, the counselor works on issues the counselor identified. The decision to terminate counseling is made either when the initial problem is no longer an issue due to the client's growth or when the problem is successfully addressed. Young Soon believes the goal of counseling can change during the process of counseling. Moving through the five stages just described may occur in a very short time and even in one session (Kim, Kim, Kim, Yoo, & Cho, 2011).

Young Soon has learned the relationship between the counselor and client is significant in the Han counseling model. Because humans are perceived as a part of the universe in this model, a counselor and client are not completely separate beings. They are interdependent since they share traits of the universe (Kim, 1982). In this model, the relationship is defined as, "you are you as well as me, and I am me as well as you" (Yoo et al., 2008, p. 8). This focus on a harmonious relationship reflects a fundamental concept of Han counseling. The model theorizes that parties in the relationship are equal and they embrace the relationship respecting each other's perspective. Because each human being is considered valuable, no one needs to change to be a better person. This assumption captures the principle of *win-win,* or *Sang Saeng* which is a term in Buddhism referring to promoting mutual interests (Yoo et al., 2008).

In the Han counseling model, when a client presents with problems, the problems become the counselor's as well as the client's. Actually, there are three parties linked with the problems: the client, counselor, and the relationship between the client and counselor. To clarify a problem, a counselor needs to explore how a client perceives the problem and how the counselor evaluates the problem. Young Soon believes when a counselor listens to the client a counselor needs to empathize with the client and display positive regard. Also, the counselor must encourage the client to assess the importance and urgency of his or her problems. After identifying the important problems, the counselor asks the client how the problem can be resolved and what the desired results of achieving resolution are. Then, the counselor evaluates the problem. In the Han counseling model, neither a pathological nor developmental perspective is used. The counselor assesses the problem as if the client has ownership of his or her life and also assesses the client's self-efficacy. Ownership of one's life is critical in this model because if someone does not experience such ownership, he or she will be controlled by past negative experiences and habits. The counselor also evaluates how a client develops and maintains relationships; how the client chooses thoughts, emotions, and behaviors; the client's self-concept; and whether the client lacks the basic need for both love and approval.

Young Soon believes in the Han model: a healthy human being has a high level of self-efficacy and good relationships with oneself, others, and the world. Self-efficacy is tied to taking ownership of one's emotions, thoughts, and behaviors. There are also responsibilities and freedom. Clients with high self-efficacy love themselves, have accurate self-concepts, and do not heavily rely on others' perceptions. The counselor employing this model examines how clients make relationships with themselves, others, and the world. The counselor assesses if the clients have right thoughts, if the clients' emotions are stable, and if the clients present adaptive behaviors (Kim et al., 2011). The clients' self-concept is also significant since it is believed one's self-image greatly impacts emotions and behaviors. Young Soon contends self-image has two aspects, ego and true self. Young Soon believes people tend to believe that the ego seen by the true self is the only self. However, she thinks there is a true self that sees the ego. Consider a person that sees himself or herself as introverted. This person has a true self that is not introverted and may be sensitive to identification as introverted because the true self is extroverted. Then, this person has both introversion and extroversion as he or she has oneself and a true self. In the Han model, a healthy individual is able to identify an ego and a true self. Another critical element of a healthy person is to choose a right thought, emotion, and behavior. A person presents different thoughts, emotions, and behaviors and selects one of them. A healthy individual chooses a positive emotion, thought, and behavior among them. Lastly, a counselor evaluates how much clients fulfill their needs for love and approval. The clients may lack love or approval from significant others or pursue love or approval excessively.

Young Soon contends that of the factors underlying clients' problems, their relationships are a primary cause of their problems, especially their emotions in their relationships. In the Han model, it is said if a person existed by oneself, there would be no problem. Because people form and remain in relationships, problems occur. Further, as relationships cause problems, the relationships need to be addressed to resolve the problems. As stated earlier, emotions in reactions to relationships are often at the root of the problem. Thus, the counselor must explore the clients' current emotions regarding their relationships rather than identify problems from the past.

The Case

JeeYoun[1] is a 45 year-old married woman who was referred for counseling to Young Soon by her friend. She lives with her husband and her children who are a boy and a girl. She is unemployed but she took financial responsibility for her family for over 10 years during her husband's education.

---

1. The client's name and some of the circumstances have been altered to protect her confidentiality.

She reported having various jobs, including serving for a short time as a teacher, until her husband became an engineer. She indicated it was difficult to work without her family's support since she needed someone to take care of her children. She also felt upset because her mother-in-law took care of other grandchildren but not hers. The client reported no issues with her husband except for parenting. Her husband lived in a different city due to his work and returned home on the weekends. The client's husband expected her to be a "perfect" mother and housewife. That is, to take care of all the household chores and responsibility to raise their children. JeeYoun pointed out her husband did not help with parenting, such as disciplining their children. During the counseling intake session, she reported having a son and daughter and conflict with her son. She also indicated that she and her family were not religious.

JeeYoun explained the mothers of her son's friends were one of her main social groups. Also, she mentioned her social status was defined by her son's academic achievement. When her son had a good academic record she reported her societal status increased and vice versa. Recently, JeeYoun expressed frustration and even shamefulness since her son was a "problem" in school and had difficulties with his academic performance. JeeYoun reported that her son's misbehavior resulted in her and her husband losing face.

JeeYoun also explained that her son's classmates at school bullied him. Her son's teacher reported he did not get along with his peers and asked inappropriate questions during class. She also was told that since he did not greet his neighbors, he was considered rude. When JeeYoun tried to discipline her son at home, he cursed and yelled at her. She expressed being very surprised at his cursing and that she was humiliated, as he had no respect for her. She emphasized that her son repeatedly asked for what he wanted until she gave in to him. She stated her daughter was different and that she was a "good" daughter. Her daughter said she could not understand her brother and she worried about his mental health.

Before starting counseling with Young Soon, JeeYoun took her son to see a psychiatrist. She revealed feeling guilty when she was told her son needed psychiatric treatment. In particular, she reported, when the psychiatrist said, "He should have come to the clinic earlier," she felt she was a failure as a mother; she felt hurt and shamed. The psychiatrist explained that her son was in a predelirium stage. JeeYoun said after quitting her job her entire identity revolved around being a mother. As a result, she felt her son's problems were her own as well. To work on all of these problems, JeeYoun attended, at no charge, 12 individual therapy sessions with Young Soon.

Contextual Conditions of Korea

Historically, in Korea, women were expected to be a mediator and provide for the physical needs of their families. Women took the entire responsibility for their household chores and parenting, and they were treated relatively poorly in the society compared to Korean men. Traditionally, married Korean women were more self-sacrificing, submissive, wise, and nurturing than men. This has changed to a degree since women started working and securing prestigious positions in the Korean society. While the modern status of Korean women has increased, they have more pressure to be good both at home and in the society. Women are required to be nurturing mothers as well as effective workers, resulting in their experiences of greater degrees of stress. Another issue resulting from modernization is the conflict that occurs between adolescents and their parents due to changing values in the Korean society (Kim, Kim, & Park, 2000; Kim, Park, & Koo, 2004). Adolescents want to have their own voice and a horizontal and independent relationship with their parents, while parents appreciate more traditional values such as filial piety and obedience toward them (Park, 2009).

JeeYoun's community is highly competitive in terms of education. Because students in her community apply for a high school based on their academic records, the parents greatly desire a better education for their children and they compete with each other. The distress linked with academic success is significant among the parents, especially the mothers, as well as the students. Since the parents greatly emphasize academics, they often neglect their relationships with one another and their children. This neglect causes additional conflicts.

Although it is a Korean indigenous counseling model, the Han model emphasizes the individual's growth. Koreans perceive a counselor as someone who assists them in solving their problems. Young Soon believes this expectation arose because of industrialization that resulted in Korea being a "speed-oriented" and competitive society. Currently, Koreans tend to rush to find the right answer or outcomes rather than appreciate the process. Young Soon is respected as an expert, professional counselor, mentor, supporter, and elder. Clients have high expectations and are even nervous to communicate with her since they consider Young Soon to be a highly educated professional. In her practice, Young Soon often is asked, "What should I do?" or "Am I doing all right?" In response, Young Soon validates her clients' desires for an answer responding, "You seem to want to know my opinion." She also asks them, "What about you?" to give power back to them in the counseling session. Young Soon believes the clients are the experts in their lives. She tells clients, "You are the one who has contemplated about your life and your issues and you are the expert on your life." Young Soon contends once clients become confident, they can solve their problems. Clients reported to Young Soon they could tell she was authentic. Moreover, Young Soon also found when a client understood and recognized her nonjudgmental attitude and display of positive regard, the client's resistance decreased and a rapport developed.

The Context

Korea is located in northeast Asia. It was divided north and south along the 38th parallel in 1945. An official South Korean government, the Republic of Korea, was founded and North Korea was formed as the Democratic People's Republic. After the Korean War in 1950, due to ideological confrontations, the division between South and North has remained. In this chapter, Korea refers to South Korea. According to the Korean Statistical Information Service (2009), in 2009, South Korea had a total population of about 48.7 million people. Koreans share one primary ethnicity and they use one Korean language, Hangeul (Korea Tourism Organization, 2011). While Korea has a foreign population because of commercial exchanges or the invasion of other countries, Korean society has shifted from a monocultural to multicultural society (Oh, 2010). The Korea Immigration Service reported, however, the foreign population in Korea as of March 2011 had increased by 1,308,743 persons.

In a survey performed by Statistics Korea in 2005, approximately 53% of Koreans reported they did not have a religion and 46.58% of Koreans indicated they had a faith. Persons who reported a religion indicated they practiced Buddhism, Protestantism, and Catholicism, 43.0%, 34.5%, and 20.6% respectively. Confucianism has had the greatest influence on traditional Korean values. It is a Chinese ethical and philosophical system that is considered a quasireligious approach to thinking and living. In Confucianism, compliance to group norms and self-regulation are appreciated, as is filial piety. Filial piety is serving one's parents with a highly respectful and proper attitude and behaviors and establishing and maintaining one's identity in reference to relationships with others. In particular, the emphasis in Confucianism on harmony in relationships has impacted how Koreans interact with each other (Kim, Kim, Seo, & Kim, 2009). The value of interdependence is reflected in Korean indigenous concepts such as *Cheong* and *We-ness* (Choi & Kim, 1998). Cheong refers to emotional bonding beyond interests. The origin of Cheong can be found among relationships between family members. When people identify Cheong, they become *we*. When individuals become *we*, they tend to make judgments by considering the closeness and the cohesiveness of group members (Choi, 2000).

Counseling in Korea

The importance of relationships is a focal point of counseling in Korea. In Korea, counseling psychology was first introduced into the schools in the form of school counseling and guidance (Kim et al., 2009). School counseling emerged due to a student-life-individuality-oriented education policy that was proposed as democratic education. This policy was a new education paradigm after the 1945 Liberation from Japan (Ryu & Park, 1998). School counseling was led first by a teacher trained in counseling psychology. Counseling professionals made great efforts to serve in school settings. There was resistance though from teachers who did not agree with employing professionals other than teachers in a school. Because violence, including bullying, became quite serious in the schools, counseling services in the school were incorporated as one form of effective solution. After passing a bill in 2007 to include coun- seling professionals in the schools, the needs of these persons in the school system became official and salient (Kim et al., 2009).

Korean counseling professionals also are affiliated with university coun- seling centers. In 1962, a student counseling center was established at Seoul National University. This center provides various services including indi- vidual and group counseling, research, and psycho-education. Currently, there are approximately 350 university counseling centers in Korea (Kim et al., 2009). Students are not charged to receive services at these centers.

Youth counseling is also prevalent in Korea. In 1991, the Korea Youth Counseling Institute (KYCI) was formed based on the Youth Foundational Law. There are 16 youth counseling centers in six cities and nine provinces. Further, there are 166 local youth counseling centers per county and dis- trict. In 2005, KYCI collaborated with local counseling centers to develop the Community Youth Safety Net (CYS-Net). This network expanded counseling from psychotherapy to outreach and advocating for youth (Koo et al., 2005). Korean youth centers do not charge adolescents for services but do receive $10 per session for adult services.

In Korea, attitudes about counseling have changed in a positive way. The value placed on saving face, however, still hinders Koreans from seeking professional counseling. Koreans prefer to share their struggles with people they are close to including friends and family members (Kim et al., 2009). Also, because Koreans appreciate collectivism, there tends to be a stigma attached to mental health issues. In particular, youth dis- play a negative perception toward counseling, as do persons of other age groups (Yoo, 1997; Yoo & Lee, 2000). While help-seeking behavior may be different from the Western culture, Korean traditional beliefs such as Buddhism are often found in counseling psychology. In fact, traditional beliefs and medicine promote the assumption that mental health pre- vents physical illness. For example, it is believed cultivating Tao through controlling the mind will promote mental and physical health. The tra- ditional religions in Korea such as Buddhism, Confucianism, and Taoism advocate pursuing self-realization or identifying the real self as an optimal status (Rhee, 1974). Finally, efforts to apply Western models of counseling in Korea and to identify Korean indigenous models continue.

The Treatment

JeeYoun presented family issues including conflicts with her son, her hus- band, and parents. She noted that she quit her work so she could commit time to raising her children. JeeYoun stated she expected her children would like her devotion to them, whereas they seemed to be overwhelmed and show resistance toward her. She reported that her son was addicted to internet games and performed poorly in school. JeeYoun explained that when she disconnected the internet at home, the conflicts between her and her son became worse. She indicated that while her husband did not engage into parenting, he blamed her for her son's problems. She expressed feeling distant from her husband, since he did not understand her, and was also experiencing conflict in her marriage. JeeYoun reported never feeling close to her mother and that family members on her husband's side seemed to look down her. Her husband's family never offered any help when she had difficulties managing work and childcare. While it is common in Korea for grandparents to assist with childcare when a husband and wife both work, recently older Koreans have focused more on their own well-being rather than helping their children and grandchildren. JeeYoun mentioned her mother-in-law did, however, take care of her other grandchildren from her daughter's side. This unfairness made her feel angry. She explained since she did not provide enough care for her children during their early childhood due to financial challenges, she felt sorry for her children. She wished she had higher tolerance toward her children. JeeYoun was surprised at her hatred toward her children during an argument. She noted feeling lost and lonely since no one seemed to understand her and she was not happy with herself.

Young Soon's perception was that JeeYoun presented a low level of self-efficacy and difficulties in relationships with others. JeeYoun had a poor self-image and she did not accept herself. She also appeared to believe her family members' judgments about her that resulted in her feeling worthless. JeeYoun had difficulties developing a good relationship with herself, others, and the world. Young Soon mentioned JeeYoun criticized herself harshly because she could not be a "perfect mother." Also, JeeYoun had few friends and felt neglected by them due to her son's academic challenges. Further, JeeYoun lacked support from her family including her husband and parents. Young Soon explained JeeYoun's low self-efficacy and struggles with relationships might stem from a lack of love and approval. In general, in the Han model, the need for approval is fulfilled by the relationship with the father and the need for love is met by the relationship with the mother. JeeYoun never felt good enough for her parents or emotionally close to her parents. Also, Young Soon observed JeeYoun chose sad or guilty emotions over positive ones. JeeYoun felt guilty because she was angry with her son. She thought she was upset because she did not like her son. However, Young Soon thought JeeYoun might be angry because she loved her son and wanted him to be successful. Young Soon's role as a counselor was to assist JeeYoun to reach her true self. When JeeYoun became close to her true self, Young Soon expected JeeYoun to have a good relationship with herself and others, and to communicate effectively.

During counseling, Young Soon first developed rapport and a trustworthy relationship with JeeYoun. As she reflected JeeYoun's emotions and empathized with her, JeeYoun learned her problem was not her own, but her and Young Soon's problem. JeeYoun stated, "[I] could tell you treated [my] problem as your own and you were eager to help [me]," and also, "You truly understand what I say, how I feel, and who I am." Further, JeeYoun said she was looking for the one who knew her and she finally met the person, Young Soon. JeeYoun also said, however, that since Young Soon reflected her like a mirror, she could not help facing her struggles. Through this relationship and interaction, JeeYoun learned how to actualize her *large self*. This self was not restricted by others, was free, was a master of her own emotions, and was able to choose a right thought and emotion, develop win-win relationships with others, and eventually become someone who was always happy and grateful for what she had.

As part of the initial counseling process, Young Soon and JeeYoun worked on setting counseling goals. As a long term goal, JeeYoun wanted to experience personal growth, accept herself, own and embrace her emotions, have a more positive self-identity, better understand her children, build a better relationship with her children, develop a more positive relationship with her other family members including her husband, reflect on her life, and make a new plan for her future. As short term goals, JeeYoun wanted to have her confidence back, perceive her children from their perspective, increase her self-efficacy for interacting with her children, change her communication style such as employing a relation-oriented conversation style, display empathetic and positive expressions, address unresolved past issues, accept and love the present, and have hope for the future. Specifically, it was expected that JeeYoun would be able to identify and express her positive emotions; control her anger toward her children; identify her deeper positive emotions; empathize with others; log and monitor her emotions, thoughts, and behaviors; engage in an empathetic conversation with her children; reinforce her children's positive characteristics; provide constructive feedback; and ultimately identify her meaning for life.

To achieve the goals reported above, Young Soon implemented several interventions connected to the Han counseling model. Before the first counseling session, during a telephone conversation, JeeYoun was asked to contemplate her past, present, and future. Young Soon learned JeeYoun was an unwanted child in her family and that as a result she developed a negative self-image. Then, Young Soon brought JeeYoun's attention to the here and now. Young Soon did not explore JeeYoun's early childhood memory excessively but rather utilized how she felt when she had a conflict with her son or when she was in a counseling session. Young Soon encouraged JeeYoun to identify and express her emotions while they interacted in a session. Young Soon described the initial session as filled with JeeYoun's venting. Young Soon believes that until the fourth session, it seemed like the prognosis for counseling succeeding was not great. During the fourth session, Young Soon challenged JeeYoun by saying she felt bored since she could not see the true JeeYoun. Young Soon pointed out that she seemed to face an invisible wall that JeeYoun constructed and maintained. Moreover, Young Soon believed that because of this, JeeYoun seemed not to be interested in communicating with her. JeeYoun appeared to be speechless in response to Young Soon's statement. When JeeYoun started expressing how she felt, she said that she was surprised, sad, anxious, and angry. JeeYoun stated, "How could a counselor treat a client so poorly?" Young Soon explained that when she empathized with JeeYoun's hurtful emotion, JeeYoun started crying with relief. Young Soon appreciated JeeYoun's honest reactions and she reinforced this expression. After this confrontation, JeeYoun was able to more effectively connect with Young Soon.

Young Soon also explored JeeYoun's similar situations outside of counseling. JeeYoun reported various emotions like worthlessness, shame, guilt, loneliness, and anger. She stated she was an unwanted child and had never felt good enough for her parents. JeeYoun noted not having support or encouragements from her husband's family either. She explained that although she was the person in charge of her family's financial and physical needs, these responsibilities were not appreciated. JeeYoun felt she was "nothing" in her family. While Young Soon empathized with JeeYoun, she also pointed out that JeeYoun tended to choose negative emotions among all her feelings. Young Soon identified emotions behind JeeYoun's surface emotions. JeeYoun admitted that although she loved her children, the consequence of disciplining them, especially her son, was conflict. She reported experiencing negative emotions toward her son.

To analyze and change JeeYoun's emotional patterns, Young Soon used two approaches, horizontal and vertical analysis. Horizontal analysis is used to identify as many feelings as possible and select a positive one among them. Vertical analysis refers to analyzing the underneath negative emotions to identify positive emotions since all persons have unlimited love in their deepest mind (Kim et al., 2011). JeeYoun revealed feeling upset and angry since her son seemed to look down on her when he misbehaved. She also reported feeling shame because her parenting might have caused her son's problems. Further, she felt guilty since she was so upset with her son. At the same time, however, she felt extremely lonely since no one in her family understood her. After JeeYoun expressed these emotions, Young Soon investigated JeeYoun's deeper emotions. JeeYoun noticed she was upset and angry because she wished her son would behave and study harder to be a success. She admitted feeling shameful due to her son's misbehavior because his success partly determined her overall success as a mother. Additionally, she noted her guilt and hatred stemmed from her love toward her son. JeeYoun expressed relief and happiness since she learned how much she loved her son in her deeper mind.

During sessions, Young Soon was a role model for how to connect with others by employing an analysis-of-communication-level approach. The analysis consists of six elements: facts and meaning, emotions, personality, hidden meanings and emotions, compliment and approval, and confrontation and feedback. Young Soon listened to JeeYoun and clarified content and the meaning of her stories. Then, Young Soon identified and empathized with JeeYoun's emotions. Next, Young Soon identified JeeYoun's personality in her story. Once Young Soon accepted JeeYoun's underneath intentions and emotions, she complimented and approved JeeYoun's meaning and emotion. Lastly, Young Soon confronted what JeeYoun missed and provided feedback. For example, Young Soon listened to descriptions of JeeYoun's typical conflicts with her children. Young Soon clarified how long JeeYoun's son played internet games and how JeeYoun restricted playing the game. She also explored and empathized with JeeYoun's emotional reactions (e.g., anger, frustration). Further, Young Soon connected JeeYoun's emotions with her personality. Young Soon believed since JeeYoun was very responsible and valued parenting compared to other parents Young Soon knew, she was more upset. She reflected JeeYoun's high motivation to educate her children. Then, Young Soon reinforced JeeYoun's positive intentions such as love and responsibility. Lastly, she evaluated JeeYoun's consequences and discussed any discrepancies between her intentions and outcomes. Young Soon and JeeYoun discussed how JeeYoun could minimize this gap and choose a positive emotion among these emotions. This was referred to as becoming a master of owning one's emotions.

Young Soon assisted JeeYoun in applying the process just described to her conversations with her son. Young Soon clarified conflict between JeeYoun and her son, empathized with JeeYoun, understood JeeYoun's personality, confronted JeeYoun's ineffective manner, and provided feedback to help JeeYoun improve her communication. Young Soon emphasized that JeeYoun needed to show empathy and appreciation first to deliver her initial intention. For example, when her son cursed her out, JeeYoun was encouraged to say, "It seems like you are really upset since you cursed me out. I know this is unusual for you to speak in this disrespectful manner and this shows how angry you are. You may be upset because I speak over and over. I know you wish I could wait more until you control yourself without my intervention. Although I understand you, the way you speak is not allowed." Young Soon explained that similar to the counseling process, JeeYoun needed to empathize first and give feedback later.

Young Soon also pointed out to JeeYoun that her communication style was not effective. Young Soon explained that JeeYoun needed to discern when it was appropriate to use a certain communication style such as fact-oriented, relation-oriented, logic-oriented, emotion-oriented, speaker's perspective-oriented, or the counterparts' perspective-oriented conversation style. In particular, Young Soon encouraged JeeYoun to use relation-oriented and counterparts' perspective-oriented conversation. Relation-oriented conversation focuses on how a conversation promotes a relationship. Let's assume that a person complains that he or she is being discriminated against. Another person could explain that he or she is being treated equally. This is a fact-oriented conversation. If another individual empathizes with the person regarding how hurtful this kind of statement could be, that is a relation-orientated conversation. Thus, when her son expresses a desire to spend more time on an internet game, JeeYoun may want to use relation and counterpart's perspective-oriented conversations to improve her relationship with him.

JeeYoun would yell at her son since she thought he ignored her and she would express her hurtful emotions. She raised her voice to show her authority but her son would become worse. Also, she admitted she did not consider her son's desire for outlets nor his frustration due to his academic struggles that made him play computer games. JeeYoun learned she needed to understand and empathize with her son first using a counterpart's perspective-oriented conversation style. JeeYoun reported she could see this vicious cycle with her son and started working on replacing a negative pattern of communication with a positive one.

JeeYoun also was encouraged to choose a right thought, emotion, and behavior as well as communication style. Young Soon explored JeeYoun's emotional reactions regarding her thoughts to distinguish a right thought and misconception. Young Soon educated JeeYoun that when she felt comfortable, her thought was a right thought, whereas when she felt uncomfortable, her thought was not right. Through this process JeeYoun also was able to identify her negative cognitive or emotional patterns.

JeeYoun learned she had compromised her identity or distanced herself from others to be a perfect mother, daughter-in-law, and wife. She reported sacrificing everything for her children. She also quit her job to concentrate on supporting her children. Further, because she wanted her children to attend a better school, she and her husband lived separately except for the weekends.

Young Soon also helped JeeYoun to understand how to dispute a wrong self-image that others might convey to her. Young Soon assisted JeeYoun in understanding that her son and husband spoke poorly about her because of their personalities and the way they interacted with her was not because of her real self. JeeYoun was able to identify her false self-image that her family members helped to shape and was able to challenge the image. An example was when her son criticized her and stated that JeeYoun was too controlling. Young Soon and JeeYoun discussed possible reasons why her son said this. One reason mentioned was that her son saw her this way because his personality was more flexible than hers. Another reason might have been he felt upset with JeeYoun, so he perceived her in a more negative way. Also, he may have said this because he wanted to have more freedom than she permitted. JeeYoun agreed he said bad things about her because he was frustrated with the situation. JeeYoun reported she felt less guilty and better about herself because of this conversation. Young Soon also assisted JeeYoun in identifying another self to see her ego. Young Soon showed JeeYoun that her true self was a great person and that she could criticize her ego.

Young Soon helped JeeYoun identify what she had accomplished. JeeYoun had done her best to nurture her children without other family members' help and she had worked hard to financially support her family. Additionally, Young Soon helped JeeYoun to identify meaning in her life, and she reinforced the value of JeeYoun's life. Young Soon believes that as a result of this intervention, JeeYoun seemed to acquire a meaning for her life, and she felt empowered.

Evaluation of the Treatment

Young Soon believes that, in general, the Han counseling model fits with a brief form of therapy. She planned approximately ten sessions with JeeYoun and intended to conduct an evaluation after about five sessions. Young Soon believes because the number of sessions was relatively short, setting a goal was significant. She terminates counseling when she and her client agree they have made sufficient progress towards accomplishing the goals.

Young Soon and JeeYoun had an evaluation at the fifth session and decided on termination at the twelfth session. During the fifth-session evaluation, Young Soon and JeeYoun discussed what she had accomplished and what she needed to work on. JeeYoun reported she learned her negative communication pattern and tendency to choose a negative emotion and thought. In the final session, Young Soon noticed JeeYoun's progress through her appearance including her facial expressions as well as her patterns of communication. Young Soon noticed JeeYoun's face was bright and peaceful and she presented herself with confidence. Young Soon believed this was a significant change because JeeYoun pursued integrity of mind, body, and spirit that was consistent with the Han counseling model. Young Soon also noticed JeeYoun was able to more effectively empathize with others. In an initial session, Young Soon thought JeeYoun seemed to talk to herself rather than to her. However, as the sessions progressed over time, JeeYoun showed empathetic and supportive responses. While JeeYoun appeared to rush to express her emotions and thoughts in the beginning of counseling, she was able to listen to others and Young Soon toward the end of their counseling relationship.

Young Soon believed it was important to specify what JeeYoun had accomplished in counseling. When JeeYoun revealed she had peace inside,

Young Soon asked her to describe this peace and the cause for the change. JeeYoun explained she was able to see how frustrated her son was when he yelled at her and cursed her. JeeYoun added she understood her son's struggles better and reacted differently by the end of counseling. JeeYoun also clearly realized how much she loved her son. This made her feel confident and relieved. She explained that while her son had not changed greatly, she could wait for his progress and connect with him better. JeeYoun also expressed a desire to learn more about parenting.

At the end of counseling, Young Soon and JeeYoun discussed her need to work on her relationship with her husband, parents, and mother-in-law. JeeYoun displayed confidence, however, that she could maintain and make progress on her positive changes. JeeYoun reported feeling proud of herself. She also admitted she previously had a poor self-image because of her high expectations and the feedback of others. Further, JeeYoun indicated her perception about her problems had changed. Now, she was not afraid of her problems and had trust and confidence to address them. She reported learning how problems help her to grow. JeeYoun stated previously she felt overwhelmed, she criticized herself, and she had high expectations. She acknowledged there were differences between having hope and high expectations. She further clarified she had hope things would get better. She intends to study horticulture and earn a certification as a florist.

Conclusion

Professional counseling arrived in Korea quite recently. Historically, Koreans held negative attitudes toward counseling, and as a result, they were not inclined to seek mental health assistance. This situation is changing as the Korean society changes. An increasing number of Koreans are entering into counseling. In this chapter, the work of a senior, highly well-respected, mental health Korean professional was highlighted as was a relatively new indigenous and innovative growth and relationship-oriented counseling model that she employs. The Han counseling model was derived from ancient Korean scriptures and other influences in the Korean society. A description of how the Korean mental health professional featured in this chapter successfully applied this model to a female client was presented. Based on clinical observations, the Han counseling model appears to be an effective brief approach to assisting Koreans with their psychological concerns. As one of only a very few indigenous models of counseling in Korea, the Han framework shows great promise in not only being beneficial to assist Korean clients but also to preserving, respecting, and promoting Korean cultural, religious, and social values, beliefs, attitudes, and behaviors. Pursuing and accomplishing these objectives is critical if the profession of counseling is to thrive and be congruent with the indigenous Korean culture and not perpetuate a United States or Euro-centric perspective of counseling and psychology.

References

Choi, D. H. (1991). *Sam-Il-Sin-Go*. Seoul, KR: HaNam.

Choi, D. H. (1996). *ChamJunGyeGyeong: Commentary on 366 Things*. Seoul, KR: Samil.

Choi, S. C. (2000). The theoretical background and practice of Korean cultural psychology: Twenty years of experiential learning through doing cultural psychology in Korea. *Korean Journal of Psychological and Social Issues. 6*(3), 25–40.

Choi, S. C., & Kim, C. W. (1998). "Shim-Cheong" psychology as a cultural psychological approach to collective meaning construction. *Korean Journal of Social and Personality Psychology, 12*(2), 79–96.

Kim, C., Kim, D., Seo, Y., & Kim, K. (2009). Professional accomplishments and current cultural challenges of counseling psychology in South Korea. In L. H. Gerstein, P. P. Heppner, S. Ægisdóttir, S-M. A. Leung, & K. L. Norsworthy. (Eds.). *International handbook of cross-cultural counseling: Cultural assumptions and practices worldwide* (pp. 173–182). Thousand Oaks, CA: Sage.

Kim, D. C. (1986). *Chun-Bu-Kyung and Dangun mythology*. Seoul, KR: Kirinwon.

Kim, G. (1982). *The principle of Han ideology*. Seoul, KR: Han Research Center.

Kim, M. J., Kim. Y. S., Kim, C.O., Yoo, D. S., & Cho, Y. S. (2011). *Han Counseling*. Seoul, KR: HakJiSa.

Kim, M. U., Kim, U., & Park, Y. S. (2000). Intergenerational differences and similarities between adolescent and adults. *Korean Journal of Social and Personality Psychology, 6*(1), 181–204.

Kim, U., Park, Y. S., & Koo, J. (2004). Adolescent culture, socialization practices, and educational achievement in Korea: Indigenous, psychological, and cultural analysis. *Korean Journal of Social and Personality Psychology, 10*, 177–209.

Koo, B., Keum, M., Kim, D., Kim, D., Nam, S., Ahn, H., Joo, Y., & Han, D. (2005). Development and intervention model for at risk-youth. Seoul, KR: National Youth Commission.

Korea Immigration Service. (2011). *Statistical resources*. Retrieved from http://www.immigration.go.kr/HP/TIMM/imm_06/imm_2011_03.jsp

Korean Statistical Information Service. (2009). *Statistical database*. Retrieved from http://www.kosis.kr/eng/index/index.jsp

Korea Tourism Organization. (2011). *Visit Korea*. Retrieved from http://english.visitkorea.or.kr/enu/index.kto

Oh, S. (2010). An exploratory study on multi-cultural education policy: Its challenges and future direction. *The Journal of Korean Educational Idea, 24*(2), 149–170.

Park, Y. K. (2009). Cultural conflicts between Korean adolescents and their parents. *Youth Culture Forum. 21*, 110–137.

Rhee, D. S. (1974). Philosophical ground-laying for psychotherapy and counseling in Korea. *Korea Journal, 14* (2), 32–37.

Ryu, J., & Park, S. (1998). Formation process of school counseling in Korea. *The Korean Journal of Counseling and Psychotherapy. 10*(1), 297–312.

Yoo, D. S. (2002). *Humanitarianism and humanity education.* Seoul: Korea Institute of Counseling.

Yoo, D. S., Kim, Y. S., & Lee, D. G. (2008). The effectiveness of a sensitivity-training program on Korean counselor trainees' locus of evaluation. Symposium conducted at the International Counseling Psychology Conference, Chicago, Illinois.

Yoo, S., & Lee, D. (2000). An exploratory study on attitudes toward seeking professional help among Koreans. *The Korean Journal of Counseling and Psychotherapy. 12*(2), 55–68.

Yoo, S. K. (1997). *Individualism-collectivism, attribution style of mental illness, depression symptomatology, and attitudes toward seeking professional help: A comparative study between Koreans and Americans* (Unpublished doctoral dissertation). University of Minnesota, Minneapolis, MN.

8 Mayan Cosmovision and Integrative Counseling

A Case Study From Guatemala

Andrés J. Consoli
María de los Ángeles Hernández Tzaquitzal
Andrea González

_____ **Introduction of the Authors**

Andrés Consoli was born and raised in Argentina, where he earned a *licenciatura* degree in clinical psychology and began his practice as a mental health professional. He moved to the United States in 1987 where he practiced as a residential counselor in a group home for autistic adults, served as a personal attendant to people with physical disabilities, worked as a bilingual counselor in a family services agency, and eventually obtained a master's degree and a doctoral degree in counseling psychology at the University of California, Santa Barbara, in 1994. He completed a research and clinical postdoctoral fellowship in the Department of Psychiatry and Behavioral Sciences at Stanford University and joined the San Francisco State University (SFSU) faculty in 1996 where he is currently a professor of counseling. Andrés has served in leadership positions with the Interamerican Society of Psychology for the past 12 years. His international work in the Americas resulted in multiple collaborations with Dr. María del

Pilar Grazioso from the Universidad del Valle de Guatemala (UVG). In the context of these collaborations Andrés met María de los Ángeles Hernández Tzaquitzal (aka, Marielos) as well as Andrea González. Both are Andrés's former students in the master's program in Counseling Psychology and Mental Health at UVG, a master's program that María del Pilar started in Guatemala in collaboration with Andrés in 2003.

Marielos, an established healer in a Mayan community of the Guatemalan countryside, also works in Guatemala City under the auspices of a non-governmental organization to help women who are survivors of trauma. Marielos, who had already earned a *licenciatura* in pedagogy and educational administration, sought further formal training in counseling through the UVG master's program. She has worked on homing in on an integrative perspective that organically brings together the Western ways of counseling and psychotherapy with the traditional ways of the Mayan cosmovision as narrated in the Popol Vuh, the sacred book of the K'iche' Maya people, *curanderismo* or indigenous healing, Catholic customs, and contemporary alternative healing methods. Andrés traveled with Marielos to her Mayan community and witnessed the respect, deference, and appreciation that villagers bestowed on her.

Andrea, an established psychotherapist in Guatemala City, earned a *licenciatura* in clinical psychology and is a graduate of the UVG master's program. She has written on the psychoanalysis field in Guatemala and has occupied several leadership positions in the mental health profession including the vice presidency of the Guatemalan Psychological Association. Andrea has worked with Andrés on several projects, most recently co-teaching the psychopathology course of the UVG master's program. Andrea has known Marielos for several years and facilitated the gathering of local information for this chapter.

The Practitioner

Marielos is known as a *curandera* (healer) in her Mayan community, that is, somebody who by virtue of her knowledge and special powers is capable of helping people in traditional, culturally congruent ways. There are many personal characteristics that make Marielos stand out. She is as approachable and unassuming as she is a patient, empathic listener. Furthermore, and at a professional level, community members gravitate to her because of the breadth of her knowledge. She integrates the traditional customs associated with a healer in her community with the Mayan cosmovision. She uses plants containing healing powers and rituals that rely on ancestral knowledge passed down through the generations. She combines traditional knowledge with more contemporary approaches such as Bach flower remedies. She also integrates the perspective of *biosalud* (literally biohealth) such as energy points or chakras with more religious, even Catholic, traditions such as praying and the use of specific types of candles depending on patients' needs.

People who seek Marielos's services are put at ease not only by her approachability and receptivity but also by her employing, at least initially, methods that are familiar to them in light of their shared cultural background. In addition, Marielos's academic credentials are a particularly attractive feature in her community, as villagers confer a high status on someone with such formal training. This is even the case when, according to Marielos, community members may not understand what the word psychologist means or what university training entails.

Overall, Marielos describes her theoretical and philosophical approach to healing as one that seeks to be integrative while empowering and strengthening the people who seek her care. She emphasizes the importance of recovering and employing traditional knowledge, such as Mayan cosmovision, and combining it with alternative healing practices as well as formal academic training. Because of her training and professional experience, Marielos recognizes that while a broad spectrum of somatic complaints brings people to consultation, what many patients really seem to need is a sensitive, perceptive listener who can address the unspoken emotional demands contained in their health-seeking behavior. She finds that it is particularly challenging to broach patients' emotional needs, though when it is done in an integrative manner, much good comes out of it and the likelihood of healing increases.

The Context

Guatemala, one of the seven countries that constitute Central America, has a population of approximately 14 million. The largest segment of the population, or about 60%, is described as *Ladina* or *Mestiza* (a heterogeneous group that has Spanish as its primary language and does not identify as indigenous), while 40% of the population are indigenous people, broadly referred to as Mayan. There are two small, nonMaya, indigenous groups that account for less than 1% of the population. One group is known as *Xinka,* and their members live mainly in Southeastern Guatemala; the other group is known as *Garífuna,* and their members are African-descended people found mainly in Guatemala's Caribbean Coast.

Guatemala is characterized by its cultural, ethnic, and linguistic diversity. While Spanish is the official language of Guatemala, there are an additional 23 recognized, indigenous languages. Social inequities also characterize Guatemala; according to the World Health Organization, 91% of the indigenous people live in poverty compared to 45% of *Ladinos/as.* The United Nations' human development index shows indigenous people lagging significantly behind *Ladinos/as* in dimensions such as life expectancy, schooling, and quality of life and facing differential barriers in accessing health care services (Hautecoeur, Zunzunegui, & Vissandjee, 2007). Guatemala's sizable share of earthquakes, hurricanes, and draughts has made these social inequities even more evident and poignant (Alejos, 2006).

The history of the Mayan people in Guatemala is a lengthy and complex one (Ekern, 1998). Unlike many other indigenous groups in Latin America, they managed to survive the Spanish conquest that began in 1523 while enduring discrimination, assimilation efforts, and exclusionary tactics (Instituto Nacional de Estadística, 2009). Following Guatemala's independence from Spain in 1821, Guatemalan Mayas continued to endure assimilation efforts, a process referred to as "Ladinization" (Falbo & de Baessa, 2006). The civil war (known as *conflicto armado* or armed conflict) that started in 1960 resulted in the death or disappearance of approximately 200,000 people and set in motion the displacement of an estimated one million Guatemalans. The civil war became, over time, a literal genocide of the Mayan people and a persecution against their Mayan culture. While it has been estimated that 90% of those killed were males, 75% of them were Mayan adult men (Berastain, 1998). Furthermore, the numerous massacres that took place in many rural, mostly Mayan communities during the civil war caused extensive social structure difficulties and engendered much distrust among Mayan people. Many Mayan groups lost their places of worship, their holidays and rituals, and some entire communities went into exile in neighboring countries, most frequently Southern Mexico. Many Mayan communities were even forbidden to wear their *traje típico* (traditional clothing), a hallmark of ethnic identity and pride.

In recent decades, efforts to rethink ethnic differences have been underway in Guatemala. In fact, new public policies have sought to value ethnic and cultural diversity (Bastos & Cumes, 2007), while educational policies created the *Escuelas Mayas* (Mayan Schools) for the purpose of advancing bilingual and intercultural education.

The peace accords of 1996 have renewed hopes for a more socially just society and have reignited the desire for Mayan social organizations and authorities (Beristain, 1998). Nevertheless, Guatemala as a country and society continues to deal with the aftermath of the civil war (Garavito, 2003). Herrera, de Jesús Mari, and Ferraz (2005) reviewed articles on mental disorder prevalence in Guatemalans published between 1962 and 2004 and concluded that there was evidence of a sizable increase of mental disorders in the population following the civil war. According to a study by the Panamerican Health Organization (Rodríguez, De la Torre, & Miranda, 2002), mental health problems, including addictions, increased during the civil war period as did people's level of frustration, hopelessness, and feelings of anomie. People were exposed to traumatic events such as torture, kidnapping, and violent deaths, which increased their sense of insecurity and fear, particularly among indigenous people. Moreover, the traditional way of transferring cultural knowledge among indigenous people from the older to the younger generation was markedly disrupted in part by the genocide and in part by the prohibitions on social gatherings imposed by the military. More recently, the displacement of large numbers of indigenous people into slum areas surrounding Guatemala City has challenged communal values such as *solidaridad* (mutual collaboration and commitment when faced with difficult, challenging, or painful situations) and *personalismo* (to treat one another with appreciation, consideration, and respect—born out of a view of one another as "you are I and I am you"). Furthermore, young Mayan refugees who went into exile in Southern Mexico during the civil war have found their homecoming experience very challenging, alternatively appropriating such experience or distancing themselves from it (Rousseau, de la Aldea, Rojas, & Foxen, 2005; Rousseau, Morales, & Foxen, 2001).

The mental health care delivery system in Guatemala is woefully underfunded, representing approximately 1% of the total health care budget. Of this 1%, the psychiatric hospital located in Guatemala City receives over 90% of the funds. This concentration of the services in the city leaves rural areas, where most Mayan people live, significantly underserved, a fact that accentuates the social inequities. In the rural areas, indigenous people are markedly underrepresented among users of the limited ambulatory mental health services (Rodríguez et al., 2007).

One possible explanation among others for such underrepresentation can be attributed to indigenous people relying more on their traditional customs that include the use of spiritual guides. These guides are consulted for and, in turn, provide advice not only on spiritual matters but also on a broad range of personal, communal, and social concerns. This is congruent with a Mayan cosmovision that does not distinguish between the sacred world and the daily living (Tovar, 2001).

To this point and according to Chávez, Pol, and Villaseñor (2005), there are six diseases in the Mayan cosmovision: *Xib'rikil* or *susto* (fright or soul loss), a condition brought about by traumatic events that results in the losing of one's soul; *Paq' ab' Chuch tat*, a condition brought about by transgressions of the social and cultural norms; *Qijalxik*, the suffering encountered by people who do not follow their vocational destiny as derived from the Mayan calendar; *Molem*, somatic manifestations of viral, parasitic, or bacterial processes that can be connected to psychosocial problems including events such as the recent civil war; *Muqu'n o pison'*, literally *buried*, a reaction among people who have deceived others; and *Moxrik*, literally *madness*, a consequence brought about by actions that should have been avoided such as envy, rancor, revenge, distrust, jealousy, violence, irresponsibility, gossip, ambition, and thievery.

There are many important resources that can help a practitioner become knowledgeable about relevant contextual dimensions in Guatemala, and familiarity with the content of these resources can shed light into the population where a given patient is immersed. We recommend sources such as the United Nations Development Program (UNDP), with country specific information and projects (www.undp.org.gt) as well as the UNDP's publications, most notably *Crecimiento con equidad: La lucha contra la pobreza en América Central (Growth with Equity: The fight against poverty in Central America)*. Though only available in Spanish, this publication is readily accessible online in its entirety at www.undp.org/latinamerica/docs/Libro_Crecimiento_con_equidad.pdf. In addition, there are periodical United Nations (UN) reports that are helpful in understanding current trends and future policies that could address such trends. We recommend *Diversidad étnico cultural: La ciudadanía en un estado plural (Cultural ethnic diversity: Citizenship in a plural state)*. This is a comprehensive report that while briefly addressing the ethnic history in Guatemala, it details matters of multiethnic justice, discrimination, and racism, among other topics. The most recent edition was published by the UN in 2006. For information that addresses what has been referred to alternatively as traditional knowledge, indigenous knowledge, traditional environmental knowledge, or traditional ecological knowledge specific to Mayan ways and that underscores important aspects of the Mayan cosmovision as it relates to its view of health and well-being, we recommend highly the following UN publication: *Raxalaj Mayab' K'aslemalil: Cosmovisión Maya Plenitud de la Vida (Raxalaj Mayab' K'aslemalil: Mayan cosmovision and life's fullness)*. Though only available in Spanish, this publication is accessible online at www.undp.org.gt/data/publicacion/Cosmovisión%20maya.pdf.

Finally, we ask the reader to keep in mind that the narratives on the practitioner, the case, and the treatment that follow are not representative of an entire country. The diversity that characterizes Guatemala, its people, and the mental health professionals who practice in the country is quite large and no single practitioner, case, or treatment could do justice to such diversity. We encourage readers to view the following narrative as a small slice of reality in an overall complex country. This slice is inherently limited by the authors' frames of reference that, in turn, have been shaped by their upbringing, education, training, and experiences. As such, the following account is humbly provided in the spirit of one sharing among others. Therefore we ask the reader to put this single case study into a larger, broader perspective so as to stay away from exoticizing dangers or tendencies.

The Case

Cintia[1] is a 17-year-old Mayan *Tz'utujil* and a high school student who was brought to Marielos by her mother. The school authorities contacted Cintia's mother following her daughter's week-long absence from school. They expressed concern for Cintia's well-being due to what they described alternatively as a "psychotic breakdown" or "dissociative process." At that time,

---

1. The client's name and some of the circumstances have been altered to protect her confidentiality.

Cintia was attending her last year in high school and was going through a particularly stressful period, feeling pressured by the school authorities to meet her sales quota of organic vegetables, a requirement of the marketing focus of her high school education. Cintia was expected to sell bags of organic vegetables door-to-door in her community, yet she found it challenging because the produce was significantly more costly than other vegetables.

What concerned school authorities the most were reports by Cintia that she had gone through some odd, recurrent, late-evening experiences. Cintia reported to them that after everybody else in her family went to sleep, she stayed up to finish her homework. Shortly after finishing, a light in her bedroom turned on on its own, she felt the presence of "images" or "figures" that tried to "grab" her, and then she experienced the pressure of a hand around her neck.

Cintia reported these experiences to her mother, a nurse at the local hospital; she had Cintia examined by health practitioners there. Cintia was told that her experiences were due to stress, most likely related to "boyfriend or friendship problems," that she needed "to take it easy," "to distract herself" with friends, and that it all would pass shortly. When Cintia did not improve, her mother sought help for her from the local Catholic priest who saw Cintia a few times. Cintia continued to experience the late evening "appearances" and her schooling began to suffer. When the school authorities contacted Cintia's mother, she decided to seek another source of care, turning to Marielos, after a recommendation by the local priest.

Cintia came to the first session looking pale, fearful, and cold to the touch, all serious signs in the Mayan cosmovision followed by Marielos. Cintia was stressed, preoccupied, and frightened. As Marielos learned more about Cintia's story, she asked about her family history, beliefs, and cultural practices. Marielos learned that Cintia's uncle, her mother's brother, died almost a year before. The cause of death was described as an accident, caused by choking on fish bones. Her uncle was a Catholic priest and Cintia was particularly close to him. Cintia's father abandoned the family when Cintia was quite young and Cintia saw her uncle as a father figure. She had two sisters. Cintia's mother's side of the family was very religious, followed Catholic traditions, yet also embraced Mayan customs.

Contextual Conditions

Cintia's community has been significantly impacted by devastating tropical storms, most recently by Hurricane Stan in 2005. Historically, the community has been impacted by decades of civil war that culminated with the peace accords of 1996. Even in the face of such challenges, the community continues to pride itself on its solidarity and the fact that people maintain active social lives that result in high-interpersonal contact.

Various Mayan groups coexist (*Kaqchikel, K'iche'* and *Tzuthuhil*) in Cintia's community; and the community itself embraces a multitude of influences including the Mayan cosmovision that include beliefs such as the presence in the world of *hacedores del mal* (evil doers or *ajitz*) and timekeepers (*ajq'ij*). By destiny, besides keeping time following the Mayan calendar, timekeepers participate in the interpretation of dreams, signals, and challenges as well as in the discernment of the divine energy that individuals possess. Cintia's community is also influenced by religious, predominantly Catholic though also Protestant, beliefs. Many other contemporary perspectives can be found in Cintia's community as well, from those that are modern but dovetail with ancestral traditions such as ecology, to others referred to collectively as *alternative healing practices* that have been incorporated into people's repertoire of help seeking and understanding of health and illness. In the midst of this sizable diversity, members of the indigenous community tend to eschew Western mental health practitioners, in part because of the distrust born out of many centuries of oppression and discrimination culminating with the civil war, and in part because of their preference for traditional Mayan ways. The mental health field has relied on informal syncretisms to bring its work into indigenous communities and on practitioners who have high credibility in the indigenous communities and who are mavericks at integrating the Mayan cosmovision with psychotherapy approaches.

Overall, health in the indigenous community is conceived as harmony between the heart, the mind, and the body that results in the person being able to work and participate in the community. Sickness is construed as an imbalance between thoughts and emotions of the spirit, the mind, and the body that gets in the way of joy, hope, and work. It can be caused by ill desire or negative thoughts, by disobedience to one's mission, by abuse of alcohol or drugs, or by disrespect of the elders.

In this context, Marielos is a recognized healer with an impressive breadth of knowledge who is comfortable with many different traditions. Furthermore, Marielos has occupied several important leadership roles in her community and people look up to her due to her extensive service.

The Treatment

Cintia's difficulties could be organized around the cultural-bound syndrome of *susto* (literally, fright) (American Psychiatric Association, 2000; Chávez et al., 2005). In the Mayan cosmovision, a *susto* is a serious condition that entails sufferers being frightened out of their spirit—referred to as soul loss—possibly losing their capacity to reason, and/or becoming vulnerable to diseases. A *susto* can be brought about by multiple causes such as bad news, an accident, or visitation by a "restless soul." In the Mayan cosmovision, restless souls are those who are not able to rest in peace, died in a traumatic manner, and are now seeking humans to aid them in achieving their final peaceful rest.

According to traditional beliefs, there are particularly vulnerable times in the day when people may be more prone to accidents, sudden deaths, or visitations by a restless soul. These times are known as *las malas horas* (literally, the bad hours) and are said to occur at midnight, at noon, and at 9:00 pm daily. Reputedly, people are most vulnerable to negative events during those times.

In the same tradition, ways to protect oneself during *las malas horas* include, but are not limited to, bathing in water blessed with certain plants, drinking tea made with similar plants, and engaging in rituals and prayers. The Mayan culture highly values the virtues of gratitude and respect. As such, one must be grateful for one's own fortunes and must honor one's ancestors by remembering them systematically if one wants to guard against the inherent vulnerability during *las malas horas*.

Yet before engaging in such conceptualizations of the presenting complaint and intervening accordingly, in the Mayan tradition, treatment is initiated by an active effort to generate in the first session a shared sense of tranquility, typically predicated on the capacity of the practitioner to enact empathy towards the patient. This empathic connection is achieved when the patient feels that the healer is a well-intended, harmless, cultivated soul. The initial goal is to put the patient at ease, something that Cintia experienced and was able to verbalize to Marielos. Meanwhile, Marielos noted that Cintia looked better towards the end of the first session, seemed more animated, and ready to participate in treatment. In this context, Marielos was able to secure from Cintia a commitment to return to classes immediately, something that Cintia did from there on, throughout treatment, and beyond.

The next phase of treatment is to inquire about the patient's beliefs and cultural frame of reference. Cintia indicated that she and her family believed in *las malas horas*, the supernatural, and a world of souls living among the living. Nevertheless, Marielos assessed for the possibility of any sexual improprieties that Cintia might have experienced at the hands of others, including her uncle. Cintia denied any such experiences or even situations that could have led to a misunderstanding.

Cintia and Marielos then discussed ways in which Cintia's experiences could be overcome. They discussed the utilization of a plant (*ruda* or rue) to clean her home and to bring to church. Meanwhile, Marielos used some of the same plant as a burnt offering. Furthermore, Cintia was to bathe in water blessed by this plant and burn some candles as a way to heal and protect her aura. Cintia and Marielos agreed to pray in their own ways to seek healing for the matter at hand. Their conversation entertained the possibility that the *susto* may have been caused by the restless soul of Cintia's uncle who died traumatically. They together considered this and agreed to some specific rituals to "send the soul on its way." As such, a mass was arranged and Cintia visited the burial grave of her uncle with her mother shortly after the mass. Furthermore, Cintia went for three consecutive Mondays to a house of worship and lit a certain type of candle for the purpose of honoring her uncle and bringing peace to his soul.

Marielos engaged Cintia in the facilitation of the mourning process. She proposed to Cintia the use of the empty chair technique, which Cintia found disconcerting initially but ultimately embraced. During these sessions, Cintia recounted her appreciation for her uncle, how much he had meant to her, and how distressing his sudden death had been to her. She felt that she had become *huérfana de padre* (orphan of father) for a second time in her short life. Cintia decided to write a letter to her uncle as a way to bring some closure to her uncle's untimely passing.

Evaluation of the Treatment

The treatment extended over six sessions and Cintia seemed to be doing significantly better. Her countenance improved markedly and she was no longer pale or cold to the touch (a troubling sign according to Mayan creation myths). Most importantly, she had not experienced any of the evening "appearances" that brought about the consultation and she attended school regularly since the first session. She did not continue treatment beyond the six sessions on her own accord, most likely due to symptom improvement. Had treatment continued, Marielos would have encouraged Cintia to focus on the pressures she experienced at school and the stress associated with them.

Marielos spoke with Cintia's mother on a few occasions. Marielos met with her during the initial session to gain an understanding of her view of her daughter's difficulties and again during the second session when Marielos sought information about any possible sexual molestation that Cintia may have experienced. Marielos also met with Cintia's mother shortly after the last session with Cintia. The mother indicated that Cintia was doing much better but that she was looking for help for herself concerning the death of her brother whom she missed dearly.

An important follow-up consisted of dialoguing with school authorities about their concerns for Cintia's well-being as well as their perspective on Cintia's struggles. With Cintia's assent and her mother's consent, Marielos made contact with the school authorities for a report on Cintia's performance. Cintia's teachers and the school principal were pleased with Cintia's progress. Based on the questions raised during their dialogue, Marielos offered to do an in-service training for the school personnel to present some more details of her approach, without discussing Cintia's treatment specifically. The training was scheduled to take place following Cintia's graduation.

Recommendations for Treatment

We would like to offer the following recommendations in the case that Cintia were to be a recent immigrant to the United States or another country. The United States is identified as a specific country because its population includes a large group of immigrants from Guatemala. We believe that a thorough understanding of Cintia's perspective on her difficulties is an important place to start the work with her. We would encourage the practitioner to first inquire about Cintia's view of her struggles. We recognize that this phase of treatment might present sizable challenges as Cintia is more likely to focus on some of the physical components of her troubles and to struggle with verbalizing the more emotional aspects of her situation. We would recommend that the practitioner facilitate a discussion about the customs, beliefs, and practices that Cintia's family follows. It would be particularly important to explore any generational differences that may exist between Cintia and her family of origin and the extent to which Cintia sees herself as identifying with the more traditional beliefs and customs. It would also be important to discuss her identification with the majority culture of the host country and any conflict she may feel between her allegiance to her culture of origin and the culture of the new country. Moreover, the experience of immigration itself is worth discussing as many immigrants from Guatemala and elsewhere from Central America have endured extremely challenging, even traumatic, events in their migratory path, not only during the journey but also once at their destination.

We would recommend that the practitioner seek the aid of a cultural broker to help elucidate some of the beliefs espoused by Cintia and her family such as *las malas horas,* the Mayan cosmovision, and the spiritual world, among others. Furthermore, the practitioner should join with Cintia in exploring culturally congruent ways that Cintia and her family believe may help address her difficulties. While the practitioner may not be able to provide all aspects of the treatment desired or sought by Cintia and her family, he or she could build community connections with whom to collaborate to address Cintia's difficulties in manners that are culturally relevant. Nonetheless, an important matter to keep in mind is the close-knit nature of many immigrant communities in the United States and other countries, a phenomenon that can make consultation difficult due to the potential compromising of confidential information and may even present particular challenges within the traditional framework of confidentiality that characterizes mental health professional practice in the Unites States and elsewhere. Another important matter to consider when working with Guatemalan immigrants in general, and particularly when the Guatemalan immigrant clients are Mayans, is the impact that the civil war may have had on them and their family. Finally, majority-culture practitioners in the United States and elsewhere should be cognizant of the unique power that they possess to help immigrants: the simple, yet profound, human capacity to welcome their immigrant patients and treat them with respect, a counterpoint to marked contextual hostilities their immigrant patients may have experienced in the host country.

References

Alejos, J. (2006). *Dialogando alteridades: Identidades y poder en Guatemala* [Dialoguing about othernesess: Identities and power in Guatemala]. Mexico: Universidad Nacional Autónoma de México.

American Psychiatric Association (2000). *Diagnostic and statistical manual of mental disorders* (4th ed., text revision). Washington, DC: Author.

Bastos, S., & Cumes, A. (2007). *Mayanización y vida cotidiana: La ideología multicultural en la sociedad guatemalteca. Volumen 1: Introducción y análisis generales* [Mayanization and daily life: Multicultural ideology in the Guatemalan society. Volume 1: Introduction and general analysis]. Guatemala: FLACSO CIRMA Cholsamaj.

Beristain, C. (1998). Guatemala, nunca más [Guatemala, Never again]. *Revista Migraciones Forzosas, 3*, 23–26.[2]

Chávez, C., Pol, F., & Villaseñor, S. (2005). Otros conceptos de enfermedad mental [Other concepts of mental illness]. *Investigación en Salud, 7*, 128–134.

Ekern, S. (1998). Las organizaciones mayas en Guatemala: Panorama y retos institucionales [Mayan organizations in Guatemala: Overview and institutional challenges]. *Mayab: Revista de la Sociedad Española de Estudios Mayas, 11*, 68–83.

Falbo, T., & de Baessa, Y. (2006). The influence of Mayan education on middle school students in Guatemala. *Cultural Diversity and Ethnic Minority Psychology, 12*, 601–614.

Garavito, M. A. (2003). *Violencia política e inhibición social: Estudio psicosocial de la realidad guatemalteca* [Political violence and social inhibition: A psychosocial study of the Guatemalan reality]. Guatemala: FLACSO-Guatemala.

Hautecoeur, M., Zunzunegui, M. V., & Vissandjee, B. (2007). Las barreras de acceso a los servicios de salud en la población indígena de Rabinal en Guatemala [Barriers to accessing health care services for the indigenous population in Rabinal, Guatemala]. *Salud Pública de México, 49*, 86–93.

Herrera, W. W., de Jesús Mari, J. J., & Ferraz, M. T. (2005). Mental disorders and the internal armed conflict in Guatemala. *Actas Españolas de Psiquiatría, 33*, 238–243.

---

2. The title in Spanish of this Journal was properly corrected starting in 2001. The Journal is a Spanish version of *Forced Migration Review* out of Oxford University. The cited article is available online, http://www.migracionesforzadas .org/pdf/RMF3/RMF3_23.pdf.

Instituto Nacional de Estadística (2009). *Marco conceptual para enfocar estadísticas de pueblos indígenas* [Conceptual framework to focus statistics of indigenous groups]. Guatemala: SEN Sistema Estadístico Nacional.

Rodríguez, J., De la Torre, A., & Miranda, C. (2002). La salud mental en situaciones de conflicto armado [Mental health in armed conflict situations]. *Biomédica, 22,* 337–346.

Rodríguez, J. J., Barrett, T., Narváez, S., Caldas, J. M., Levav, I., & Saxena, S. (2007). Sistemas de salud mental en El Salvador, Guatemala y Nicaragua: Resultados de una evaluación mediante el WHO-AIMS [Mental health systems in El Salvador, Guatemala, and Nicaragua: Results of a WHO-AIMS evaluation]. *Revista Panamericana de Salud Pública, 22,* 348–357.

Rousseau, C., de la Aldea, E., Rojas, M., & Foxen, P. (2005). After the NGO's departure: Changing memory strategies of young Mayan refugees who returned to Guatemala as a community. *Anthropology & Medicine, 12,* 1–19.

Rousseau, C., Morales, M., & Foxen, P. (2001). Going home: Giving voice to memory strategies of young Mayan refugees who returned to Guatemala as a community. *Culture, Medicine & Psychiatry, 25,* 135–168.

Tovar, M. (2001). *Perfil de los pueblos: Maya, Garífuna y Xinka de Guatemala. Proyecto de Asistencia Técnica Regional* [Peoples' profiles: Maya, Garífuna and Xinka of Guatemala. Regional Technical Assistance Project]. Guatemala: World Bank & Guatemalan Ministry of Culture and Sports (MICUDE).

Authors' Note

Andrés J. Consoli, PhD, is professor of counseling at San Francisco State University and may be reached at consoli@sfsu.edu. María de los Ángeles Hernández Tzaquitzal is a healer and psychotherapist in Guatemala and may be reached at hernandeztzaquitzal@yahoo.com. Andrea González is in private practice in Guatemala City and may be reached at yeya.gonzalez@gmail.com.

9

Disaster Counseling

A Haitian Family Case Post January 12, 2010 Earthquake

Gargi Roysircar

Introduction of the Author

My name is Gargi Roysircar and I am a professor of clinical psychology, founding director of the Multicultural Center for Research and Practice, and a licensed psychologist at Antioch University New England. An immigrant from India, I have lived in the United States for 32 years, first as a "green card holder" and then as a naturalized citizen. In my extended family now, we have three distinct immigrant generations, and I am familiar with adapting to different worldviews within our generational systems. I am a Hindu, a woman, a feminist, and am bilingual in English and my native language, Bengali. I am familiar with other languages like Hindi, Marathi, and French but do not claim proficiency in them. My practice in the United States and internationally is essentially cross-cultural because my individual clients, group clients, consumers, or psychology trainees have heritages different from mine. My professional work, as presented in the following pages, is as diverse as I am.

Since 2005, I have participated in disaster mental health response in Haiti, tsunami-affected Southern India, Hurricanes Katrina- and Rita-affected communities, responder organizations in the United States Gulf Coast, and in Southern African orphanages for HIV/AIDS-infected and affected children and women. I have provided psychoeducational programming in flood-ravaged Villahermosa, Tabasco, in Southern Mexico. I train my volunteer doctoral student response teams in disaster trauma, culture-centered response skills specific to a community, and in responder self-care. My student team and I focus on our role in the ecosystem and advocate within the micro as well as macro larger systems to facilitate healing and resilience in destroyed communities. We call ourselves Disaster Shakti, which means empowerment, mental strength, hardiness, and resilience in several languages of India. Disaster Shakti means empowerment in the face of a disaster.

International disaster counseling aligns with my university's value of community action for a just and sustainable society and its credo "The world needs you now"; it is in keeping with our value of inclusiveness of people of diverse backgrounds. The learning activities and goals of international disaster counseling operationalize our university's vision and core values of quality education, inclusiveness, social justice, experiential learning, and socially engaged citizenship. In honor of my disaster-response mental health outreach, I was awarded in 2011 with my university's first Horace Mann Spirit of Service award.

The Practitioner

Traditionally, psychologists serve clients who have been individually assessed and diagnosed, for example, for trauma. We do not provide community-level interventions for grief and loss responses that do not constitute ameliorating individual psychopathology. Yet, the roles of mental health providers in the 21st century are expanding and, as a corollary, our practice has become more diverse. Disaster mental health broadens the scope of conventional practice when it ameliorates the effects of disasters at the community level. We participate in community resilience and rebuilding services. Social justice is practiced in vulnerable communities, settings where disproportionate numbers of poor people, women, children, and orphans are often the most tragically affected by a disaster. In far too many cases, the people affected by trauma are in developing countries. These communities have the fewest resources for rebuilding.

Disaster response, at the same time, is mental health work that utilizes mental health professionals' unique skill sets. Active listening, empathy, and relational skills are paramount. What will help the overly angry or depressed parent take control, express his or her needs clearly, and return to parenting children? Is the seemingly unemotional person in the medical patient line in a tent city experiencing shock? Other nontherapist volunteers lack the skills to listen and evaluate a survivor's emotional state in the way a mental health professional can. In addition, our skills in assessing and managing group behavior, assisting in decision making, and normalizing reactions are invaluable. Recognizing and preventing staff burnout or compassion fatigue in a relief organization and providing consultation to parents, employers, school officials, and emergency services, as needed, are opportunities to use one's psychological training.

Disaster Shakti members give ourselves significant leeway to identify unmet needs in the survivor community and to apply our professional background. We provide crisis intervention, psychological first aid, stress-management services and skills training, grief and loss counseling to adults and children, and brief structured therapy for those who present with trauma problems and posttraumatic stress disorder (Roysircar, Podkova, & Pignatiello, in press). Those interested in school services can attend a meeting with local school administrators to discuss ways to prepare students, families, and teachers as schools reopen upon recovery. Others can be enlisted to do self-care training with emergency staff (Roysircar, 2008) or advocate for disenfranchised residents with other assistance agencies, such as hospitals and food distribution centers. It is difficult, if not impossible, to describe an average day of disaster response practice, as each disaster operation is different. Using one's psychological training to quickly and thoroughly assess a changing situation, to always wear one's psychological cap, even when the task does not appear psychological in nature, is a hallmark of doing disaster mental health work (Bowman & Roysircar, 2011).

Use of Integrative and Flexible Practices

While my student volunteer team and I practice professional psychology, we have learned to relinquish prior roles, identities, and preconceived notions of what "should be." Our skill set is not limited to psychology and includes structural, sociological, economic, and sociopolitical analyses. Thus, Disaster Shakti's service is genuinely interdisciplinary and ecological in focus. We adapt to the nature of the emergency as well as to the cultural, political, and geographic contexts in which a disaster has occurred. We know to avoid a clinical response along rigid agency party lines and we know not to enter into theoretical wars (Roysircar, 2009b).

Developing a Resilience Framework to Understand Survivors and Responders

Because Disaster Shakti's philosophy is about resilience and return to mental health, we avoid pathologizing and, instead, emphasize normal reactions to abnormal situations (Ryff & Singer, 2002). We believe that disaster psychology needs to move away from identifying psychopathology. Solely assessing risk factors does not provide a complete picture of a person's functioning; a valid picture of functioning also requires assessing positive psychology and protective mental health factors (Roysircar, 2011b). We hold the view that effective traditional or native healing mechanisms may be underappreciated when we diagnose as psychopathology normal reactions to trauma and stigmatize mental health struggles. We view mental health interventions as supplemental to existing informal support networks for community resilience building.

Self-Assessment for Preparedness

Before getting involved in disaster work, Disaster Shakti members ask our-selves several questions to do self-assessment and assess our preparedness. Prior to accompanying a missionary group to earthquake-ravaged Haiti, we researched the horrific conditions of mental health care in Port-au-Prince. We learned that inside this city's earthquake-cracked psychiatric hospital, a schizophrenic man lay naked on a concrete floor, caked in dust. Other patients, padlocked in tiny cells, clutched the bars and howled for atten-tion. Feces clotted the gutter outside a ward where urine pooled under metal cots without mattresses. As is common with disasters in areas of low socioeconomic status, Haiti's January 12, 2010, earthquake exposed and amplified the severe inadequacies of its mental health resources. This inad-equacy occurred when such services were most needed. It is worth noting that before the earthquake, there were only a handful of psychiatrists in all of Haiti, indicating that mental health resources were vastly insufficient prior to the national crisis. Reading such information was daunting for the majority of the Disaster Shakti members. Only two volunteers self-assessed that they had the skill and the will to serve as therapists in a clinic, which to date had only received medical and construction volunteers.

Rural Setting in Haiti

We served in a medical clinic run by a Protestant organization, Partners in Development (PID), whose headquarters is located in a second-floor suite in Ipswich, Massachusetts. Its Haiti clinic, serving since 1990, is located in Blanchard, the poorest of poor communities outside Port au Prince and assists as well those living in tent villages of Canaan and Damien. Mobile units primarily serve prenatal care in tent villages that do not have access to medical care. The Blanchard clinic provides care for high blood pressure, diabetes, eye care, and postnatal care to about 50,000 people every year. PID has a similar operation in Guatemala.

Disaster Shakti members paid a little over $1000 each to PID for our air-fare, boarding, and lodging to serve as volunteers in Haiti. In addition to our own suitcase, each of us carried a bag of Haitian-returning-from-the-United States-proportions filled with medicines. We were provided these bags by PID at Logan airport. In one week, the clinic with one Haitian doctor and American nurses, who are like Florence Nightingale in their selfless dedica-tion, as well as local community health workers served 800 patients. Each day from 8.00 a.m. to 5.00 p.m. for two weeks, I provided crisis management and grief/loss counseling and self-care education to individuals, families, couples, and groups of women and girls. I served approximately 100 clients altogether. One other counselor and a pastor did similar counseling work. We were the first mental health practitioners to serve since the PID clinic opened in 1990.

Our counseling spaces were created under blue tarps tied to trees, one concrete wall, and clothes lines. A Disaster Shakti student commented, "We counselors often fill our counseling spaces with objects that comfort, compel, or distract in some fashion. Two chairs (or three) and some shade seem just right now and right to the point." The student described so aptly how counseling can be done in open spaces in Haiti. People in the compound knew to give us psychological privacy and not to listen in or gawk at us. This phenomenon is common in crowded living spaces of poor societies. In Haiti, a whole family of 15 may live in one room or tent. While there is little physical privacy in such arrangements, there is psychological privacy and interpersonal respect. Roosters, hens, chicks, baby lambs, beautiful white doves, two mangy dogs, lots of insects, and fruit-laden coconut, mango, jackfruit, and papaya trees were our clinic decorations—attention getting in their own natural ways. Roosters crowed here at all times, with wake-up calls at 2:00 a.m.

Our translators were young men for whom there was no public college to attend in the earthquake's aftermath, and they could not afford the tuition of Catholic colleges in Port-au-Prince. The translators were self-taught English-speakers and, at their own initiative, they had downloaded medical and psychiatric information from WebMD (www.webmd.com) from the clinic's only computer, and they walked around the compound carrying wads of such printed information reading and memorizing like medical students. I trained the translators for half a day on their roles with the counselor and client (Bradford & Munoz, 1993; British Psychological Society, 2008; Panigua, 2005; Perez-Foster, 1998), and they were quick learners. The translators did not work with their own family members in counseling but rather provided educational materials on such matters as stress and muscle relaxation. The young men provided the best translation services that I have experienced in my international work.

The conditions in Haiti were desperate, in every sense of the word, six months after the earthquake. Large-scale disaster response organizations had not met with success. The smaller missionary-led or philanthropic organizations that had located themselves within tent villages and cities were doing effective work and were accepted by the local people. Larger organizations like Doctors Without Borders, American Red Cross International, and World Health Organization had pulled out their operations. It was my privilege and honor to share in the lives of Haitian women, men, youth, and children, whose spirit to survive as well as their resilience, good humor, hard work, and faith in God, despite constant hunger, unemployment, and no infrastructure to speak of, made me a stronger and hopeful therapist. As the 4th of July came around, I cherished the rights, privileges, safety, police protection, and opportunities that the United States had granted me, an immigrant, which the Haitian government in contrast had neglected for its own native-born poor people. Armed guards with guns protected our compound at night. I never saw them and only learned about their presence at an emergency meeting of leaders, which included me. We were informed that some intruders had scaled our compound's high walls topped with sharp glass edges and that these intruders were apprehended by the guards. We were then asked to communicate this information to our teams and discuss methods of concealment and escape should our guest house be attacked at night.

Outcome Assessment

As participant researchers in our action research, Disaster Shakti trainees were made aware of their various disaster-related cognitions and affect, sources of resilience, positive characteristics, level of multicultural sensitivity, and (for those of European American descent) their White racial identity and privilege interfacing with people of color and indigent survivors (Roysircar, 2011a; Roysircar & Brodeur, 2010; Roysircar, Brodeur, & Irigoyen, 2008). In their daily journaling at a disaster site, Shakti members, including me, pondered on their self-reflective practice.

The Case

It was 8:00 a.m. and already large numbers of men, women, and children were standing outside the padlocked PID gates. As the compound iron gates were opened, people filed in, forming long lines. *Tap tap* trucks unloaded more people into the compound. Many came on foot, walking four hours to get to the clinic, and they would return on foot for another four hours. But the majority of the people were from the four nearby tent villages. Now and then, out on the dirt broken road, a bed frame moved slowly toward the gate, with a bearer at each corner and a very sick patient on the mattress. No one was turned away, and each patient was given a ticket. They were the poor, pregnant, maimed, and blind. By 9:00 a.m., a crowd of about 40 waited in the clinic's lobby which had a well-maintained indoor garden. Some sat on benches clutching their tickets, and others milled around. There were children everywhere. There were two examining rooms, one room for the pharmacy, and one room for Mr. Essen, who dispensed donated shoes, school supplies, and coloring books to children. I wished he could also give bags of beans and rice because all were hungry, but PID did not provide food.

I was fresh and ready to receive my first client at 9:00 a.m. I saw a young man do the Haitian hand slap, the back of one hand into the palm of the other and ask my translator questions. The translator brought him into my blue tarp tent and said, "Doktè Gargi, this person wants to know what type of doctor you are. I told him 'doctor of mind.' Then he asked if you were a sorcerer, and I said a good sorcerer." I explained to Ti Jean, my translator, "A counselor is a healer; please tell him that." The family case that follows is a composite case of clients that I served in Blanchard. No particular individual or family can be identified, and all names have been changed.

Ti Ofa, the client, said that he was feeling down and the past few days his right ear was also hurting bad. I thought an earache seemed like a medical problem. I told him that he needed to tell the doctor and the nurse about his earache. Ti Ofa said he brought his mother to see the doctor and that he would tell the doctor about his earache. He said he needed to get back into the line for his mother and that he would come back.

An hour or so later, Ti Ofa was sitting on a fallen tree trunk across from my tent, smiling at me. I was between clients and asked him to come in. Ti Ofa showed me a small prescription bottle and opened it. He said that the doctor had pulled bed bugs out of his ear, and Ti Ofa asked the doctor to place the extracted bugs in a bottle so that he could show these to Doktè Gargi. Ti Ofa then said that he wanted his sisters and their children to meet the new *doktè*. He waved his hand to a group of women hovering nearby, and they hesitantly came toward us carrying babies in their arms and pulling other children by the hand. As we greeted each other, I met Serena and Didi, the two older sisters, and Yolande and Ti Fifi, the two younger sisters. I gave energy chocolate bars to the children who had sticklike limbs and asked whether I could hold a baby. As this was happening, the director of PID, Gale Hull, hurried into the tent and said that she needed to speak to me alone. We stepped outside and Gale said the mother of the family had stage-four stomach cancer and requested that I help the mother and her daughters and son understand the seriousness of her illness and make plans for the future. Ti Ofa went to get his mother, who in pain, was bent at the waist and leaned on Ti Ofa as she slowly moved toward the tent. Her legs were very swollen and she breathed heavily. We helped *mami mwen* (my mother) to lie on the bench in my tent. Mami moaned loudly, "li fe-m mal, mwen grangou," translated by Ti Jean, "it hurts, I'm hungry." I immediately gave mami and her daughters and son energy bars. As they and the children ate with small bites, I thought that Haitians had adapted themselves to starvation, but counseling may be more effective if the family had some nourishment.

During the earthquake, a wall fell on the father as he was resting after work and he was killed when the whole house crumbled. His wife and four daughters, with their babies and children, were at the marketplace selling their wares, while his son idled outside. All belongings and materials were lost. In their relocation to a tent village, the husbands and boyfriends of the daughters either ran off with other women or simply disappeared. The daughters said that the ill will of other women and neighbors caused a curse that took away the males in their family, that is, their father and their partners. Their brother, who was not perceived as strong or impressive as a male, was spared. The mother raised herself and stared accusingly at the third daughter. Yolande said, "mami mwen hates me. I feel ashamed." In fact, mami believed that this daughter's partner, who quarreled often with her father, sent the earthquake that killed her father.

I reflected to the mother not that the supernatural does not exist, but that I know that sorcery did not cause the earthquake. In line with the guidelines for psychological first aid for disasters, I gave information about the earthquake to the family as well as information about the development and progress of cancer. Gradually, mami softened, but it would take a long time to fully reconcile her with surviving male members of her family, while her husband was less fortunate. She asserted that only she at her age (50) and with her life experience could manage the household. It would take her several months to reconcile that she would no longer have the strength and capacity to wield the power she did as *mami mwen* with her many children, grandchildren, and extended relatives.

Ti Fifi, one of the younger sisters, hardly spoke. She sat on the bench with a despondent, defeated look, her head held low, and her arms cradling a baby. Cumulative crises occurring at once (i.e., the loss of a strong male figure in the household, an ailing mother, her boyfriend's abandonment, and no house to live in) were likely very painful. Ti Fifi appeared to be suffering silently, which warranted closer examination. Serena, the oldest commented, "We have problems, but we're not dead as yet."

Faith in mental health, medicine, and prayers, while contradictory, prevailed. Mami asked, while we were in the middle of our conversation, that we join hands and say a prayer. In turn, I asked Reverend Nate, who was a pastoral counselor, to lead us in a prayer circle. We met for counseling the rest of the day and each session, all of which occurred over the span of that day for several hours, ended with us standing up, holding hands while Reverend Nate said a prayer that the Alcante family's new learning in counseling and efforts to renew family life would be blessed. Each session began with progressive muscle relaxation training to help the family members cope with their reported stress reactions of headaches, neckaches, muscle tension, insomnia, and racing hearts. The family described obsessive thoughts that the earthquake would happen again and reported that they even felt their bodies and chairs shaking. They compulsively counted their few things and referred to what appeared to be auditory hallucinations of crackling and crashing sounds. The family cursed the demons that had possessed their bodies.

Remembering the Haitian proverb, "Beyond mountains there are mountains," I told myself I could not ignore the complexity of perspectives in my understanding of my Haitian clients' many realities. This was an epiphany for me. Was I going to refuse treatment to people who thought that death, loss, grief, cancer, and physical stress came from sorcery?

The Context

Haiti, the poorest country in the Western Hemisphere, has struggled for decades with poverty; oppression; death from tuberculosis, HIV/AIDS, malaria; and death of children from measles. On January 12, 2010, a 7.0 magnitude earthquake that lasted just a few seconds and was a shallow earthquake destroyed the capital of Haiti, Port-au-Prince (United States Geological Survey [USGS], 2010). The Haitian government reported that an estimated 210,000 people were killed, and about 700,000 civilians were homeless or displaced (United States Agency for International Development, 2010). The USGS (2010) reported worse numbers: an estimated 222,570 were killed, 300,000 injured, 1.3 million displaced, 97,294 houses destroyed, and 188,383 houses damaged in the Port-au-Prince area. Many parts of Haiti are still in reconstruction today, and the process to rebuild has been difficult (United States Department of State, 2011). In October 2010 the Haiti Ministry of Health announced a cholera outbreak throughout the country. Nearly 50,000 people sought medical help, of whom 19,646 cases were confirmed as having cholera. By November 26, 1,600 Haitians had died from cholera (Guzman, 2010; Republique d'Haiti Ministère de la Santé Publique, 2011).

The native language of Haiti is Creole, while Haitians with higher levels of education also speak French (Coupeau, 2008). Many Haitians are very optimistic, hardworking, and strongly believe, despite all odds, in their ability to control their personal situations and future (Desrosiers & St. Fleurose, 2002).

History

Haitians have a history of resilience and optimism that is worthy of narration by a Homer, a Tolstoy, or a Tolkien. Christopher Columbus landed on the island that he named Hispaniola, and the extermination of Arawak Indians then ensued. The island was divided between France and Spain, leaving the French in possession of the island's western third where they created an immensely lucrative and gruesome slave trade, in which one third of every new shipment of West African slaves died within three years. In 1791, Haitian slaves staged the only successful slave revolt in the history of the Americas (Coupeau, 2008). Not even Napoleon and 40,000 French troops could put down the revolt. At last, in 1804 Haiti was created and was Latin America's first independent nation and the world's first Black republic. Haitian Creole is, in essence, a romance language, derived from French and, in some of its phonetic habits and grammatical structures, also clearly West African. It is unique to Haiti, expressive and born out of grim reality. The French masters deliberately separated slaves who spoke the same language, and the slaves fashioned their own tongue. Many

Haitians are proud of this history and view it as a strength of their culture (Desrosiers & St. Fleurose, 2002).

But independence was followed by nearly 200 years of misrule, aided and abetted by foreign powers, such as France and the United States. From 1915 to 1934, United States marines ran the country and trained and developed the Haitian army after the United States took charge of Haiti under President Woodrow Wilson. Francois Duvalier, the infamous Papa Doc, ruled the country with liberal use of terror from 1957 until his death in 1971. His reign continued by his son Baby Doc with the same proclivity for murdering political enemies and for stealing and misappropriating foreign aid, of which the United States was aware and did not stop.

Baby Doc proclaimed himself "president for life." So influential were the Duvaliers that when Mother Teresa visited Haiti in 1981, she affectionately praised the dictator, said that she learned a lesson in humility from the dictator's wife, and marveled at the closeness of the first lady to her people; in actuality, Baby Doc's wife was widely hated by Haitians, and she had looted millions from the Haitian treasury for her worldwide shopping sprees (Kidder, 2004) The streets of Port au Prince were patrolled by Duvaliers's Praetorian guard, the men in dark glasses, the "*tontons macoutes,*" named for a mythical bogeyman, Uncle Sack, who stuffed bad children into his bag (Kidder, 2004).

In 1986, soon after Baby Doc was forced to leave Haiti, there followed what dissident Haitians called Duvalierism without Duvalier, with the Haitian army generally taking on the dictatorial role. In Port-au-Prince, political demonstrations were rampant, which included a *kouri,* literally a run or a stampede of people, followed in close pursuit by large Haitian army trucks with mounted guns. Shots were fired at fleeing protestors. For many years to come, the smell of burning tires, military blockades, and massacres were the abiding odor of Haiti (Kidder, 2004). At the center of the popular revolt were Catholic churches in the ruined countryside and in Port-au-Prince slums and in one of the latter presided the priest Jean-Bertrand Aristide. In 1990, foreign observers that included President Jimmy Carter certified the results of a national election; 67% of the votes were for Aristide, whose government had the most popular support of any in the world. In 1991 the Haitian army deposed Aristide.

The three years of military rule resembled a war. The United Nations estimated that about 8,000 people were killed by the Haitian army and its paramilitaries. Thousands of boat people drowned while trying to get away to the United States. Other boatloads of refugees, fleeing the poverty and violence of Haiti, managed to reach Florida and were promptly sent back by United States immigration officials. The treatment of Haitians was different from that of Cubans, who were accepted by the United States reportedly because they were political and not economic refugees. Aristide was reinstated in mid-October 1994, and he was encouraged and economically supported by President Clinton, who had a personal interest in Haiti and had spent his honeymoon there with his wife, now Secretary of State Hillary Clinton, when they were young lawyers. Aristide was re-elected in late 2000, but the economic conditions of the country grew worse and worse with declining foreign aid. After the January 12, 2010, earthquake, governmental help was nonexistent and the ruling party was in disarray. Politicians jockeyed for power and re-election, with the former dictator Baby Doc, as well as Aristide, exiled in South Africa, making re-entries into Haiti, and the current president, Rene Preval, wanting to remain in power at the end of his term of office. After two rounds of voting, November election results were announced in December, which led to riots. Despite the Provisional Election Council sanctioning the election, protests continued, and almost two thirds of the candidates called for the election to be annulled, alleging fraud and that many voters were refused ballots. Protests continued in Port-au-Prince and Gonaives, with barricades in the streets and the airport closed. Port-au-Prince had four consecutive days of protests after the election results, while the results were supported by the United Nations and the United States. It's to be noted that President Obama tried to stop Aristide, a former United States ally, from returning to Haiti during the election campaign. Despite momentous upheavals, Haitians have not lost their culture.

Religion

Before the introduction of Christianity with the arrival of Columbus, Haitians practiced the religion of *Voudou* (also known as Voudoun or Voodoo). Voodou is an African spiritual belief system that involves the supernatural and good and evil spirits, called *Iwas*. Iwas must be respected and honored through special ceremonies, usually performed with the aid of a *Hougan* (male priest) or *Mambo* (female priestess) (Nicolas, DeSilva, Grey, & Gonzalez-Eastep, 2006). Contrary to popular belief, this spiritual practice rarely includes cursing others, though Haitians may believe that mental or physical illness as well as any sort of misfortune is due to being cursed by an unhappy Iwas or someone that is jealous of them. While members of the lower economic and social classes are the most likely to engage in Voudou practices in comparison to their more affluent counterparts, most Haitians today are Roman Catholic and Protestant (Charters, Taylor, Jackson, & Lincoln, 2008). Many Haitians incorporate Voudou practices into Christian beliefs and believe Catholic saints and biblical characters can also represent Iwas. According to an old saying, perhaps less true now than formerly, Haiti was 90% Catholic and 100% Voodou (Desrosiers & St. Fleurose, 2002).

In the Haitian countryside, there is a distinction between belief in sorcery and the practice of Voodou (Kidder, 2004). Not every peasant practices the indigenous religion of Voodou, but virtually everyone, including Catholics, Protestants, and Voodouists, believe in the reality of *maji*, or sorcery (Kidder, 2004). For many people around Blanchard, where we worked, maji spells sent by enemies are the deep cause of many illnesses. And many people believe that doctors, like all good Voodou priests, know how to contend with magi.

Haitian Beliefs About Death and Grief

It is necessary to understand the spiritual beliefs and background of Haitian culture to foster understanding and empathy towards Haitian clients in counseling. Knowledge of these beliefs helps counselors facilitate the use of spirituality as a strength during bereavement. Those that practice Voudou believe in an afterlife and that every person has two souls: the big angel (*gros bon ange*), which is a universal life force; and the small angel (*ti bon ange*), which is the individual soul. It is believed these souls remain near the body for several days following death but can be at risk for capture by evil spirits. During this time, the family gathers to perform rituals and mourn the dead (Métraux, 1972). Response to death is often accompanied by physical displays of emotion, including wailing and crying to mourn the loss (Laguerre, 1984). At the end of this period, a Hougan or Mambo engages in rituals to free the soul from its body. It is believed the soul becomes an Iwas as well to protect and watch over the family (Métraux, 1972).

The death of a loved one may be easier to accept when the cause seems explainable, while acceptance may be more difficult for clients that believe their loved ones died as result of a curse or an angry Iwas. This belief often leads to significant feelings of guilt, anger, and distress. The surviving family members may feel compelled to engage in spiritual practices to appease the angry Iwas and be at peace with the loss (Eisenbruch, 1984).

Haitian memorial rituals vary based on the individual family and economic status. As many Haitians are Catholic and Protestant, they may engage in practices similar to those of people in the Unites States who have the same faiths. Others may have incorporated Voudou beliefs into Christian beliefs and may express variations in their beliefs regarding the afterlife. Until the funeral, Haitians may conduct a wake every evening to celebrate and remember the life of the deceased. A death in the family often elicits the involvement of all extended family members (Laguerre, 1984).

Mental Health of Haitians

While Haitians who have suffered loss may go through the Kubler-Ross's stages of grief, that is, denial, anger, bargaining, depression, and acceptance, they may manifest these reactions differently and, therefore, they're difficult to identify. Haitians often have a holistic view of health and describe health as a variety of physical and psychosocial factors, much like the concept of wellness. However, Haitians do not perceive physical or mental symptoms as an illness unless they are incapacitating (Laguerre, 1984). Haitians may not take notice of symptoms of depression, anxiety, or grief until they get to the point that they can no longer work or engage in daily responsibilities. As they pay little attention to mental health, these symptoms often manifest in somatic symptoms. Haitians that engage in Voudou may believe mental illness is the result of being cursed or not engaging in spiritual rituals to respect Iwas (Desrosiers & St. Fleurose, 2002).

While there are many culture-specific illnesses in Haiti, the most relevant illness in the postearthquake context is *Se'izisman*. Se'izisman is a nearly catatonic state in which the individual becomes disoriented and unable to function. Haitians believe this is caused by viewing a traumatic event, being informed of a significant loss, or dealing with a difficult situation (Nicolas et al., 2006). It is believed Se'izisman causes a rush of blood to the head and puts the sufferer at higher risk for further health problems or even suffocation or death (Laguerre, 1984). This may manifest in every individual differently, and one person may experience Se'izisman for an hour while another experiences it for several days. The proper response to this altered state is caretaking of the individual, including emotional support and physical support, such as massage, herbal remedies, and consumption of particular foods (Nicolas et al., 2006). It is helpful for counselors working with Haitians to be aware of the signs and symptoms of Se'izisman as well as the culturally acceptable helping responses.

Suggestions for Counselors

These suggestions are based on the available limited literature for working with Haitian American clients, which perspective I maintained in my disaster counseling in Haiti. It should be remembered that the suggestions may or may not apply to clients based on their individuality, local community factors, education, and social class.

- The counselor should use a strength-based approach, as optimism and resilience are a theme in Haitian culture that can be beneficial during counseling sessions (Desrosiers & St. Fleurose, 2002).
- Family members can be important assets in counseling and if possible, should be involved in the treatment process (Nicolas et al., 2006). This is especially true if the whole family is coping with loss and struggling with acceptance, as the family can work together on how they will cope and grieve in a productive and healthy manner.
- The counselor should align with the client, even if the client's beliefs are different from the counselor's personal beliefs. For example, Haitians may believe the misfortunes of the earthquake are due to evil spirits or curses (Desrosiers & St. Fleurose, 2002). By aligning with

Haitians, the counselor can help them work through the grief in their own manner. For example, it may be helpful for the client to engage in a spiritual ritual to respect and remember loved ones and feel that they can move on without the risk of further misfortune.

- It may be helpful to adapt traditional counseling methods of managing grief and frame them as a spiritual exercise for the clients. Examples of such exercises may include helping the client create a memory box of significant objects that remind them of their lost family members or encouraging the client to write a message to the deceased and attach it to a helium balloon to be released in a ceremonial manner (Roysircar, 2008). Both of these activities can be framed as a ritual to respect and honor those lost while also helping the client work through and address his or her grief.

- As Haitian Americans are often hardworking and dedicated to supporting family members, counselors can help Haitian clients understand that unmanaged symptoms of grief can cause them to be less productive and reduce their ability to provide for their family. Thus, the solution is to work through this grief in counseling (Desrosiers & St. Fleurose, 2002).

- Consulting with and involving spiritual healers in the Haitian American community can be helpful in working with this population (Nicolas et al., 2006). Healers may have suggestions on how to integrate traditional Haitian spiritual practices into counseling as well as help clients to trust mental health services.

- It may be helpful to collaborate interprofessionally with other service providers, including medical doctors and nurses, that can link clients with resources to increase wellness and facilitate the grief process, including medical care, support systems in the community, financial resources, and toys and clothes for children. For example, clinicians may be able to work directly with physicians to manage physical ailments and clarify whether physical symptoms are related to psychological distress (Desrosiers & St. Fleurose, 2002).

- Counselors should actively engage clients and have a concrete plan of action at the end of each the session because Haitian clients want to feel that time spent in counseling is productive. (Desrosiers & St. Fleurose, 2002).

- Ethically, counselors must be sure they have effectively communicated issues of confidentiality with their clients. Such communication should be able to be translated into their language in both oral and written form. Family members should not be used as translators; instead a trained translator should be utilized.

- Last, counselors should adhere to the multicultural counseling competencies, including an awareness of their own cultural values and biases, awareness of the client's worldview, and an awareness of culturally appropriate interventions strategies (Roysircar, Arredondo, Fuertes, Ponterotto, & Toporek, 2003).

The Treatment

The treatment for the Alcante family was a combination of addressing the grieving process, management of family crises, and relaxation training.

The Grieving Process

First, the focus was on the grieving process. The family was grieving different types of losses: the death of their father, abandonment by the husbands and boyfriends of the four sisters, the mother, Ruth's advanced stage of cancer, the destruction of their house, and the loss of the life they knew before the earthquake. I was especially concerned about the family's phenomenological experience of these major losses. Conceptualizing the Alcante family's losses in terms of Kubler-Ross's stages of grief (Kubler–Ross & Kessler, 2005) was a place to start.

Depression, according to Kubler-Ross and Kessler (2005), is conceptualized as an appropriate reaction to a loss, rather than pathology. The Alcante family had empty feelings associated with their various losses. While in counseling might have been the first time that they felt the sorrow of losing so much. At that stage, the grieving family could "take stock" of their losses as they had finally slowed down enough six months after the earthquake (Kubler-Ross & Kessler, 2005). In addition, their mother's recent cancer diagnosis was an opening to really experience some of the associated feelings of loss.

The family was depressed because they were coming to terms with the reality of their new life in the aftermath of the earthquake: their father was gone, the mother was terminally ill, and the sisters' husbands and boyfriends might not return. The final stage, acceptance, had to be characterized by realizing the reality of losses. At that stage, grieving persons form a new relationship with the deceased, which might allay depressed feelings. I assisted the family with forming new spiritual and positive connections with their deceased father, their mother's new role as a patient, and with their life prior to the earthquake.

In addition to an individual response to loss, grief is a social loss, which varies considerably across cultures (Koenig & Davies, 2003). It was necessary for me to "step outside" of my own two cultures, Asian Indian and American, in order to generate an understanding of how to work with the Alcante family, according to their grief. First, I educated myself on how grief and loss are handled in the Haitian culture. I tried to understand how death is understood and handled in the Alcante family. What were the traditions and practices of the siblings for mourning? Did all siblings mourn similarly or differently? What did the surviving extended family members do to grieve their father's loss and respond to their mother's cancer? I explored how they imagined their departed father's ongoing spiritual and protective relationship with them and their mother's new relationship with them in her widow-hood and present illness. Could the family, all affected by the crisis, take several journeys down memory lane to rediscover and tell stories about their deceased father, about their missing husbands and boyfriends, and about their mother before her widowhood and her present illness?

Acquiring knowledge about Haitian mourning rituals had not fully prepared me to work with the Alcante family. I had to also understand differences within groups, in the event that the Alcante family did not sub-scribe to bereavement norms associated with a particular Haitian religious group. While the Alcante family members were practicing Catholics, they also said that the devil had swallowed their father. I assessed differences at the individual level by asking: "Can you help me understand how you and your family mourned over your father's death?" Koenig and Davies (2003) encourage clinicians to make use of outside resources, such as community or religious leaders or family members, when working with clients whose culture is unfamiliar to the practitioner in order to understand grief and loss in line with the client's culture. In this particular case, I asked whether the Alcante family had the opportunity to be involved in a Haitian local community like in their resettlement tent village for support and spiritual sustenance during the past six months of mourning. I also aimed to learn, understand, and adopt a particular language associated with grief and loss by asking the Alcante family what terms resonated with their current state of grief. Doing so demonstrated linguistic sensitivity to the Alcante family's bereavement process.

As a young woman in the Alcante family, there were specific roles Ti Fifi needed to fulfill. However, her despondent and melancholic behavior was an obstacle to her contributions to the family. I realized I needed to be aware of how her behavior was perceived within her culture. From a psychological standpoint, Ti Fifi was suffering from depression. The recent events affected her differently than her family members. However, in Haitian culture, depression is called *discouragement,* and is not viewed as a mental illness. Instead, it is interpreted as a generally debilitating state caused by malnutrition, worry, or a curse. Haitian culture does not view depression as a viable illness and believes that an individual has control over how it affects him or her (Desrosiers & St. Fleurose, 2002). Discussing the psychological impact that discouragement could have on Ti Fifi and her family was a paramount task. In this process, it was crucial to not only give credence to cultural mores but also to stress the impact that discouragement could have on the functioning of the Alcante family.

The Alcante family experienced loss at multiple levels. In fact, the loss of their father symbolized their many other personal losses and the future possible loss of their mother. Meaning-making occurred according to variations at each contextual level: the loss of their life in Haiti at the meso level and the loss of their many identities as mother, wife, daughter, son, and lover at the micro and interpersonal levels. If the family's meaning-making of their losses had involved deep sorrow or anger, I might have used interventions that explored negative emotionality, from which the family could learn to enhance their well-being. But, this process was not necessary as the Alcante family was coping in a pragmatic and functional manner. They came to the Blanchard clinic weekly with their mother, they went to the market place to sell their wares, they washed their clothes dressed neatly, they lived altogether in one tent, and they made friends in their camp. Interventions for the Alcante family's grief and loss issues demonstrated sensitivity to their steps of survival. A lack of awareness of cultural responses to loss could have led to misinterpretation of depression reactions, failure to offer appropriate support and assistance perceived as helpful, and might have even offended the grieving persons and created a barrier to their openness to receiving treatment.

Postmodern Family Therapy

Postmodernism poses many challenges to the perspective of modernism that has dominated American psychology since the late 19th century. While modernism suggests the existence of an objective reality that can be sought, observed, and known with a sense of empirical certainty, postmodernism emphasizes the subjective nature of individual realities and reconceptualizes knowledge and truth as a matter of perspective as well as individual and local narratives. The postmodern perspective has had an increasing influence on the field of psychotherapy since the 1990s, especially in family therapy.

Therapist and Client Roles. From a postmodern perspective, the therapist and client are reconceptualized as having equally valid perspectives. The therapist is viewed as having expertise in the process of therapy, while the client is viewed as having expertise in his or her many personal realities and narratives. However, neither of these forms of expertise is to be valued over the other. Instead, "the therapist introduces an idea, but does not necessarily believe that people should follow it" (Becvar & Becvar, 2009, p. 92).

Language. Postmodernism places a great emphasis on the use of language. Becvar and Becvar (2009) write,

> In the process of socialization, we learn to speak in accepted ways and simultaneously to adopt the shared values and ideology of our language system. Thus, our words express the conventions, the symbols, and the metaphors of our particular group. And we cannot speak in a language separate from that of our community. (p. 91)

As a result, the attitudes, values, and biases of the Alcante family's reference groups were inherent in the way the Alcante family came to describe, explain, and account for their world and themselves. For instance, the sisters spoke about other jealous women and girls stealing away their husbands and boyfriends and, at the same time, they blamed reigning evil spirits for the earthquake, their father's death, the disappearance of their partners, and for their mother's illness. The mother agreed with their narratives and insisted that they should say prayers with her. The brother commented that he had seen his brothers-in-law with other women.

Postmodern family therapy seeks to bring family members into dialogue with one another in such a way that they understand the stories each family member uses to construct his or her reality. As therapy progresses, family members help each other, with the support of their therapist, to construct new stories and thus a new reality. The goal for this reconstruction of the family's reality is to free them from the problem-laden stories they brought to therapy at the start.

The brother, who was the youngest, said that he did not participate in family responsibilities and that he did not feel confident that he could make any contribution to the family. The sisters' stories were that the brother remained at home while they worked as street vendors, and he took care of their children; they believed he could learn from the sisters to keep things picked up and do some food preparation. The brother joined the sisters' stories that he was not like other adolescent boys who roamed the camps, were thieves, and looked at girls. Yet, he said he was lazy, and the sisters joked that they could change that easily.

The Use of Questions. Much of postmodern family therapy is based on the therapist asking the client questions, but the therapist must always pose these questions in a tentative manner. There are three major categories of questions: (1) the miracle question, (2) the exception-finding question, and (3) the scaling question (Kaslow, Dausch, & Ciliano, 2005).

The miracle question I asked the Alcante siblings was to explain how they would know when their problem was gone, as if they woke up and a positive maji had solved the problem. They were asked to explain how the world would look, feel, and be different after the problem-solving miracle. The goal of this type of question was to help the Alcante siblings find their own solutions to their problems by focusing on solutions and outcomes, rather than staying stuck on the problem. The siblings all said that they would create in their tent an atmosphere of rest and peace for their mother, share her leadership among themselves, and work hard to bring home more money and food. The brother said that he would take care of their mother like he took care of his sisters' children while his sisters were selling in the market. They all said that they would go to church daily in addition to Sunday service to pray for their mother's health and their departed father. They said they would come to the Blanchard clinic regularly to check on their health and their children's health.

The exception-finding question I asked the Alcante siblings was to think about times when the problem of losses and their mother's illness did not influence them. Clients often focus so much on the ways that the problem is affecting their lives that they fail to notice when the problem is absent. Such exceptions can provide clues to clients about solutions that have not been tried yet. The Alcante siblings said that they all felt very good on Sunday mornings when they, their mother, and their children dressed nicely and went to church. There the priest's long sermon resonating through loudspeakers and the congregation's jubilant singing was motivational, and they felt blessed like they were before the earthquake when the family was intact and their mother in good health. After the main service, they joined small prayer and educational groups in the church annex, as they did before the earthquake.

The scaling question, for example, asked Ruth, the mother, to rate on a scale of one to ten how severe the cancer and family leadership problems were at various points during the course of counseling. I wanted to allow Ruth to focus on small instances of progress as she was resistant to accepting her diagnosis. I asked Ruth, who rated the family leadership problem as a four, what it might take to move to a five in the upcoming session when the children would discuss how they would share her family responsibilities and her caretaking, including bringing her to the clinic for regular checkups. Ruth rated the problem of accepting her illness at a one at the beginning of the session, when she argued energetically that her children could not manage the family without her authority and experience. When we joined hands and followed Reverend Nate in his prayers for blessings for the family and for me, the therapist, Ruth's rating reached a five for both problems. This scaling allowed the mother to home in on small steps toward larger goals of problem resolution (Kaslow et al., 2005).

Lakes, Lopez, and Garro (2006) discuss a method of intervention in which the therapist and client co-construct a narrative based on a shared worldview. This acknowledgement of different therapist and client worldviews and attempts at integrating these differences into a joint narrative (like saying a prayer together, being focused on the family's well-being, and the sick mother still honored as the head of the household), was very important in this family case. Given that Haitians see therapists from different cultures, especially from the United States, therapists and clients need to work together to define problems and search for solutions that are in-line with the shared understanding of the clients' world co-constructed by the therapist and the client.

Zimmerman and Dickerson (1994) take a similar approach to family therapy, using narrative approaches to work with adolescents (in the present case the brother, the youngest child) and families (the mother and the sisters). The authors suggest that problems between parents and adolescents are often caused by different narratives in the different subsystems.

For instance, the parents may have had a story for the future of their child since the child's birth or even earlier. As the adolescent develops and begins to author his own narrative, he may begin to develop a story for himself that is very different from his parents' projected story for his life. For instance, Ruth wanted her son to have a small business as his father had, but the son wanted to remain at home with his nephews and nieces.

Helping parents and their adolescents articulate their individual narratives and then share them with each other is suggested as an intervention that can help families gain a greater understanding of the way these differing narratives are contributing to what has become a problem in their lives. As families develop a greater appreciation for the impact of these narratives on the lives of each family member, they may be able to develop a dialogue that allows them to re-author their stories in a more congruent way.

Once treatment with the Alcante family began, the goals of therapy were identified. These entailed establishment or clarification of a hierarchical structure, in which Ruth, the ailing mother, was clearly the authority. Another goal relevant to this case was the formation or maintenance of clear boundaries and roles within the sibling subsystem, with the brother as the outlier being pulled into the sibling subsystem. This family presented with slightly rigid boundaries, especially in the case of mother as authoritarian and adult children as subservient. This traditional boundary was functional before the earthquake, but postearthquake, with changes in the family composition and the mother's health status, the boundary needed re-alignment. The goal here was to increase interaction between Ruth, the mother, and the younger sisters and the brother who may have been more neglected or at times forgotten and even threatened. Parental boundary re-alignment increased nurturance and the perception of safety and support for the marginalized children. In large families, such as the Alcante family, especially in the case of a single parent–run family of a large size, it may be necessary for older children to take on parental roles in order for the family to operate effectively. This flexibility in roles is not a problem in and of itself, but it can become an issue if the child is required to carry out tasks that are above his or her ability level, such as Ruth's expectation of her son in this case. Furthermore, problems may arise if the child in the caretaking role is not validated or supported by the parent (Becvar & Becvar, 2009). Ruth was reluctant to share her charge with her older daughters. Even though in pain, lying on a bench, she shouted her commands to her grown daughters or said that we needed to join her in prayers.

Mother Subsystem. The mother subsystem operates functionally through influence of a hierarchical structure; the mother must exist in a role of authority and power in contrast to the children, who must understand that their parent takes a superior role within the context of the family (Becvar & Becvar, 2009). The children's acceptance of the parent as an authority figure is crucial for their acceptance and ability to interact appropriately in other social situations in which authority is unequal, as in the context of interacting with teachers, law enforcement, doctors, the church, and other people in jurisdictional roles. This had been the traditional organization in the Alcante family likely through the generations but more pertinent to the living members in the past 30 years. But then roles changed. The father was dead and the mother terminally ill. The two older daughters needed to take over the household while still respecting and honoring the mother's presence and seeking her consultation and advice.

Sibling Subsystem. This system refers to the interaction, communication, and relationships between the children of the family. Through these interactions, the children learn how to appropriately and effectively play, compete, and compromise with peers outside of the family in the context of the greater social system. The children that comprise the sibling subsystem also learn to come together to challenge the parental subsystem. In the healthy family, the sibling subsystem is aware of its position relative to the parental subsystem. However, in the present case, the two older sisters moved into the parental subsystem to join their mother and share her authority and responsibilities.

Progressive Muscle Relaxation and Diaphragmatic Breathing

Because the Alcante family reported many physical symptoms of stress, I thought the most culturally congruent method of treatment would be progressive muscle relaxation. The family responded to relaxation training naturally, and it appeared to have had more impact on individual members than other methods of counseling described above. Progressive muscle relaxation involves intentional relaxation of the muscles that tighten under stress by using slow, deep breaths that help the parasympathetic nervous system lower blood pressure and heart rate. Progressive muscle relaxation lowers arousal levels so it becomes more challenging to the body to manifest later physical symptoms of stress and anxiety, so it can be preventative of physical stress reactions (Wehrenberg, 2008). In addition, progressive muscle relaxation can directly treat muscle aches and stiffness that accompany reactions to anxiety-provoking situations (Wehrenberg, 2008).

I told the Alcante family that the primary goal of progressive muscle relaxation was to relax all of the muscle groups in 10 to 15 minutes. I added relaxing imagery into the process, referring to the Blanchard compound's towering palm trees; shorter ones laden with jackfruit, papaya, and mangoes; the bougainvillea flowering shrubs: and the bright blue sky with patches of clouds. I expected that focusing on local imagery would assist those family members who had difficulties focusing on their bodily reactions.

The first step involved finding a comfortable place to sit in a relaxed position, keeping the neck upright. Next, I instructed them to close their eyes in order to focus on a specific group of muscles. Once a muscle group was identified, the next step involved tensing, holding, and then relaxing each muscle. We did this rotation three times for each muscle group.

Diaphragmatic breathing involves taking slow deep breaths that fill the stomach and allow for the release of tension from the body (Wehrenberg, 2008). As noted by Wehrenberg (2008), diaphragmatic breathing appears to naturally occur while engaging in progressive muscle relaxation. I encouraged the Alcante family members to notice how they breathed during the muscle relaxation process. Diaphragmatic breathing motivates the parasympathetic nervous system to calm systems which are activated during stress, such as the neuroendocrine system (Wehrenberg, 2008). I found the local imagery to be useful in pairing relaxation with diaphragmatic breathing.

Evaluation of the Treatment

Although the Haitian population has been in need of mental health resources since and prior to the earthquake, a very low percentage actually use mental health services. Haitians have little knowledge of how to seek out mental health services or manage the bureaucratic barriers they may be confronted with (Portes, Kyle, & Eaton, 1992). Haitian clients will most likely be referred to counseling by other health professionals, and they may lack an understanding of the benefits of counseling. They may also be cautious of counseling services based on poor treatment by other community or government agencies. I acquired knowledge about the Haitian culture of origin and its history and politics so that I could render culturally sensitive disaster counseling following the January 12, 2010, earthquake. That the Alcante family willingly utilized my services for nearly a whole day suggested that they liked me and what I had to offer. Since I was doing crisis management work, I stabilized them and did not plan to see them again unless an emergency arose. We were in the same neighborhood and the mobile units did not report further problems in the family while I was still there. I wonder whether my counseling continues to affect them positively one year after Ti Ofa came to my tent with an ear ache.

On the other hand, I do research on Disaster Shakti volunteers so as to improve our future disaster services. One study (Roysircar, 2011a) examined the relationship of disaster responders' characteristics with resilience. The characteristics were positive or negative thoughts and feelings about responder work, a sense of personal accomplishment, multicultural awareness, multicultural relationship, solitude pleasant events, and a collectivistic worldview. Disaster Shakti volunteers in Haiti were included in this study. Other Disaster Shakti volunteer teams provided psychological first aid and listened to hurricane survivors in the United States Gulf Coast and psychosocial programming for HIV/AIDS-infected and -affected orphans and women in South Africa and Botswana as well as for flood-displaced residents of Villahermosa, Mexico. Participants were two cohorts: disaster volunteers (n = 20) and nonvolunteers (n = 20). In addition to experiencing response work, the volunteers received training for a semester prior to responding, while the nonvolunteers did not receive such training. The two groups were matched on age, sex, disciplinary education, social class, and self-reported race, ethnicity, or national origin. Each group self-administered the self-report measures four times over a two-week period of response work. Multivariate repeated measures dependent t-tests showed that volunteers had higher levels of personal accomplishment (p<.01 d=.15, a medium effect size), multicultural awareness (p<.001 d=.58, a large effect size), and multicultural relationship (p <.05 d=.17, a medium effect size), after Bonferonni adjustment was performed. Nonvolunteers used solitude pleasant events more frequently than volunteers (p <.001 d=-2.5, a large effect size). Multiple regression analysis found that personal accomplishment, multicultural relationship, solitude pleasant events, and groups (volunteers versus nonvolunteers) were each significant predictors of resilience for a total variance of R^2 =.54. This quantitative part of Disaster Shakti's program evaluation has led Shakti volunteers to receive training in yoga, diaphragmatic breathing, muscle relaxation, and pleasant imagery. Volunteers' low scores in solitude pleasant events suggested that they needed to practice emotional self-care when deployed.

Conclusion

While I may know how to adapt mainstream therapies to be culturally sensitive and how to practice the multicultural competence of awareness of my own and my client's worldview, these alone are not sufficient for carrying out effective counseling. There is the issue of essential common factors, including therapist empathy and warmth, the ability to effectively implement interventions along relationship-building lines, and the capacity to form a working alliance with a client who is culturally different from the therapist (Roysircar, 2009a; Roysircar & Gill, 2010). My cross-cultural empathy was comprised of a really felt and expressed affect with the Alcante family who lived in earthquake-cracked Blanchard, Haiti; perspective-taking of their diverse cultural, spiritual, economic, political, and healthcare contexts; and individual and family empowerment that bridged gaps that exist in bereavement, family, and cognitive-behavioral interventions.

References

Becvar, D. S., & Becvar, R. J. (2009). *Family therapy: A systemic integration.* Boston, MA: Allyn & Bacon.

Bowman, S., & Roysircar, G. (2011). Training and practice in trauma, catastrophes, and disaster counseling. *The Counseling Psychologist. 39*(8), 1160–1181

Bradford, D. T., & Munoz A. (1993). Translation in bilingual therapy. *Professional Psychology: Research and Practice, 24, 52–61.*

British Psychological Society, Professional Practice Board (2008). *Working with interpreters in health settings: Guidelines for psychologists.* London, UK: Author.

Charters, L. M., Taylor, R. J., Jackson, J. S., & Lincoln, K. D. (2008). Religious coping among African Americans, Caribbean Blacks and non-Hispanic whites. *Journal of Community Psychology, 36*(3), 371–386.

Coupeau, S. (2008). *The History of Haiti.* Westport, CT: Greenwood Press.

Desrosiers, A., & St. Fleurose, S. (2002). Treating Haitian patients: Key cultural aspects. *American Journal of Psychotherapy, 56*(4), 508–521.

Eisenbruch, M. (1984). Cross-cultural aspects of bereavement: Ethnic and cultural variations in the development of bereavement practices. *Culture, Medicine and Psychiatry, 8*(4), 315–347.

Guzman, J. (2010, November 26). Médecins San Frontieres struggles against cholera in Haiti. *Demotix, News by You.* Retrieved from http://www.demotix .com>North America>Haiti>Port-au-Prince

Kaslow, N. J., Dausch, B. M., & Ciliano, M. (2005). Family therapies. In A. Gurman & S. Messer (Eds.). *Essential psychotherapies.* (2nd ed., pp. 400–462). New York, NY: Guilford.

Kidder, T. (2004). *Mountains beyond mountains.* New York, NY: Random House.

Koenig, B., & Davies, E. (2003). Cultural dimensions of care at life's end for children and their families. In M. J. Field & R. E. Behrman (Eds.), *When children die: Improving palliative and end of life care for children and their families* (pp. 509–552). Washington, DC: National Academies Press.

Kubler–Ross, E., & Kessler, D. (2005). *On grief and grieving: Finding the meaning of grief through the five stages of loss.* New York, NY: Scribner.

Laguerre, M. S. (1984). Health beliefs and practices. In *American Odyssey: Haitians in the United States* (pp. 109–129). Ithaca, NY: Cornell University Press.

Lakes, K., López, S. R., & Garro, L. C. (2006). Cultural competence and psychotherapy: Applying anthropologically informed conceptions of culture. *Psychotherapy: Theory, Research, Training, 43*(4), 380–396.

Métraux, A., translated by Hugo Charteris. (1972). *Voodoo in Haiti.* New York, NY: Schocken Books.

Nicolas, G., DeSilva, A. M., Grey, K. S., & Gonzalez-Eastep, D. (2006). Using a multicultural lens to understand illnesses among Haitians living in America. *Professional Psychology: Research and Practice, 37*(6), 702–707.

Panigua, F. A. (2005). *Assessing and treating culturally diverse clients: A practical guide* (2nd ed.). Thousand Oaks, CA: SAGE.

Perez-Foster, R. (1998). *The power of language in the clinical process: Assessing and treating the bilingual client.* Lanham, MD: Jason Aronson.

Portes, A., Kyle, D., & Eaton, W. W. (1992). Mental illness and help-seeking behavior among Mariel Cuban and Haitian refugees in South Florida. *Journal of Health and Social Behavior, 33*(4), 283–298.

Republique d'Haiti Ministère de la Santé. (February 4, 2011). *Publique et de la Population* Retrieved from http://www.mspp.gouv.ht/site/index .php?option=com_content&view=article&id=57&Itemid=1

Roysircar, G. (2008). *Building community resilience in Mississippi: Self-care for disaster response workers and caregivers* (Grantor: Foundation of the Mid-South in partnership with the America Red Cross). Keene, NH: Antioch University New England, Multicultural Center for Research and Practice.

Roysircar, G. (2009a). Evidence-based practice and its implications for culturally sensitive treatment. *Journal of Multicultural Counseling and Development,* 37(2), 66–82.

Roysircar, G. (2009b). *Therapist, heal society and thyself: Social justice advocacy in disaster response work.* Keynote presented at the National Multicultural Summit and Conference, New Orleans, LA.

Roysircar, G. (2011a). Disaster response competencies of responders: A pilot study. Paper presented at the annual conference of the American Psychological Association, Washington, DC.

Roysircar, G. (2011b). Foreword: Positive psychology, Eastern religions, and multicultural psychology. In E. Chang & C. Downey (Eds.), *Handbook of race and development in mental health* (pp. vii–xi). New York, NY: Springer.

Roysircar, G., Arredondo, P., Fuertes, J. N., Ponterotto, J. G., & Toporek, R. L. (2003). *Multicultural counseling competencies: Association for Multicultural Counseling and Development.* Alexandria, VA: AMCD.

Roysircar, G., & Brodeur, M. (2010). *Assessment of resilience and its protective factors in disaster outreach volunteers.* Paper presented at the annual conference of the American Psychological Association, San Diego, CA.

Roysircar, G. Brodeur, M., & Irigoyen, J. (2008). *Self-care and resilience of disaster response volunteers: Outcome Evaluations.* Paper presented at the Annual conference of the American Psychological Association, Boston, MA.

Roysircar, G., & Gill, P. (2010). Cultural encapsulation and decapsulation of therapist trainees. In M. M. Leach, & J. Aten (Eds.). *Culture and the therapeutic process: A guide for mental health professionals* (pp.157–180). New York, NY: Routledge/Taylor & Francis.

Roysircar, G., Podkova, M., & Pignatiello, V. (in press). Crisis intervention, social class, and counseling: Macrolevel disaster effects. In W. M. Liu (Ed.), *The Oxford Handbook of social class in counseling.* New York, NY: Oxford University Press.

Ryff, C. D., & Singer, B. (2002). Flourishing under fire: Resilience as a prototype of challenged thriving. In C. L. M. Keyes & J. Haidt (Eds.), *Flourishing: Positive psychology and the life well-lived* (pp. 15–36). Washington, DC: APA.

United States Agency for International Development. (2010). *Fact Sheet #33, HAITI-Earthquake*. Retrieved from http://haiti.usaid.gov/our_work/ humanitarian_assistance/disaster_assistance/countries/haiti/template/fs_sr/ fy2010/haiti_eq_fs33_02–14–2010.pdf

United States Geological Survey. (2010). *Earthquake Statistics.* Retrieved from http://earthquake.usgs.gov/earthquakes/recenteqsww/Quakes/us2010rja6.php

United States Department of State, Bureau of Western Hemisphere Affairs. (2011). *Haiti: One year later.* Retrieved from http://www.state.gov/s/hsc/rls/154255 .htm

Wehrenberg, M. (2008). *The 10 best-ever anxiety management techniques: Understanding how your brain makes you anxious and what you can do to change it.* New York, NY: W. W. Norton.

Zimmerman, J. L., & Dickerson, V. C. (1994). Using a narrative metaphor: Implications for theory and clinical practice. *Family Process, 33*(1), 233–245.

10

Mr. Paul T

A Black Man in America

Camille A. Clay
Chalmer E. Thompson

_____ **Introduction**

The following is a case description of Mr. T, a mature African American man who lives and works in Washington, DC, the capital of the United States of America. In addition to presenting details about Mr. T and his treatment, we share information about the U.S. context and an overview of some of the research pertaining to the quality of life for Black Americans in general and for those living in urban U.S. settings like Washington, DC, in particular. The terms Black American and African American are used interchangeably in this chapter.

We, the authors, are two Black women who professionally have been influenced and mentored by many people from a range of racial, ethnic, nationalistic, and ideological backgrounds. We are grateful to these men and women for molding us as practitioners and scholars. We pay homage in this chapter to the Black male scholars who contributed to our thinking and practice and do so by making prominent the extent of talent that too often goes unnoticed. To denote the contributions by Black men, we have placed asterisks beside their names. These are the authors who, to the best of our knowledge, have identified themselves as African-descended (e.g., African American, Afro-Caribbean, etc.).

We begin the chapter by recounting an experience we have both shared on occasion when we interact with Black men. "How're you doing?" is a common passing greeting in the United States, not necessarily (or usually) meant to invite the person being asked to reveal much more than an "I'm well," "Pretty good," or "All right." The response also is typically positive, even when the person being asked is not really feeling especially positive that day or at that moment (Althen & Bennett, 2011). When we ask some of our Black male family members or companions, "How're you doing?" some respond, "Hey, I'm a Black man in America," or some close facsimile of this statement. To us, this rather unique response brings attention to the fatiguing burden they endure as targets of depersonalizing stereotypes of Black men as ne'er-do-wells, malcontents, and inherent criminals. Their responses even appear to be a plea to listen closely, to call attention to a condition worthy of pause and reflection, and to offer a reassuring remark. According to Kenneth Clark,* a former president of the American Psychological Association, along with others (Carter*, 2007; Parham*, 2009; Pieterse* & Carter*, 2007; Utsey*, Bolden*, & Brown*, 2001; White* & Parham*, 1990), racism, as well as all forms of structural inequality, levies a toll on individual psyches. Together these forces contribute to shaping the U.S. landscape (Bell*, 2008; West*, 2001), intermingle into our professions unless we deliberately and forcefully resist them, and permeate to and from other nations. It is imperative that we in the mental health professions understand the gravity of these burdens on individuals and societies (Cesaire*, 2001; Fanon*, 1967; Watts*, Williams*, & Jagers*, 2003). We hope to convey the gravity of these forces in this chapter as well as an understanding of the legacy of resistance to oppression, which also contributes to the cultural and sociopolitical landscape of this nation (e.g., Hilliard*, 1997; Kelley* & Lewis*, 2005; Robinson*, 2001).

The Authors and the Practitioner _____

Chalmer E. Thompson

I am a counseling psychologist whose career has been primarily academic. I have several publications based mainly on the topic of racial identity development theory, the professional development of psychologists, and psychotherapy process (that is, what occurs over the course of therapy in every session, particularly as therapist and client make sense of the role of oppression in the life of the client). I have worked at four universities as a professor, including the University of California at Santa Barbara, the University of Southern California, and Indiana University at Bloomington. In past years, I have occasionally seen clients and I continually supervise students in their counseling work. My move to the urban campus of Indiana University in 2006 was for the purpose of helping develop a social justice–oriented academic program, which entailed partnering with local urban school districts and making efforts to translate and test the premises of racial identity theory to professional development and social activism. I completed a bachelor's degree in psychology from Howard University in Washington, DC, and a master's degree in clinical psychology from Towson State University, where I met Dr. Clay, my co-author. Then in 1988, I received a doctoral degree in counseling psychology from the University of Maryland, College Park. I am fellow of the American Psychological Association (APA) in two divisions, Society for Counseling Psychology (Division 17) and Society for the Study of Ethnic Minority Psychology (Division 45); and a member of two other divisions, Peace Psychology (Division 48) and International Psychology (Division 52). I have also taught professional development courses to faculty members who come from a range of disciplines at Kyambogo University (KYU) in Kampala, Uganda, and have consulted with KYU lecturers in developing master and doctoral level curriculum in psychology. This partnership is ongoing. I have a special interest in the role of peace studies in the advancement of psychological theory, research, and practice.

As I mentioned earlier, I met Dr. Clay when I was in graduate school; this was nearly 30 years ago. I was then and still am now very impressed with her. I have met many practicing psychologists and have even referred people to a few of them, but with the vast majority of people who come to me and who live in the Washington, DC, area, my referrals have been exclusively to her. I make these referrals because Dr. Clay's manner is quite calming and her persona is one of quiet self-confidence. She listens well and shows eagerness in learning about people as people—their interests and joys. She speaks knowledgeably about issues of race and culture and has comfortably kneaded this knowledge into her work. To be sure, not every person she sees in therapy presents with or even has concerns about race or culture. But because her understanding about these matters is well entrenched and mature along a developmental continuum of racial identity (see Thompson & Carter*, 1997), her racial and ethnic knowledge is merely what informs her about each person, nothing more and nothing less than the myriad other forces that shape people and contexts. This knowledge also necessarily informs her of who she is and of the dynamics that characterize relationships, organizations, and communities.

I am convinced that the qualities I observe in her are the sort that are fundamental to exceptional psychological practice. She is concerned with the soul or spirit of her clients (see Parham*, 2009). My observations are based not only on the interactions between the two of us but also on my observations of her interactions with others. I was beginning my education as a psychotherapist myself when we first met, and I sensed from my first contacts with her that she exhibited skills I wanted to emulate. She displays an uncompromising regard for all people. She makes an effort to know people. I was aware that she also possessed an armament of strategies that are primarily cognitive-behavioral and that have helped her accomplish what she and her *client*, the term she uses for the people who seek her services, wanted to accomplish in the therapy. I also know she uses sound, ethical judgment in her relationships with her clients. I have referred several people to Dr. Clay and in each case, the people I've referred have reported back to me that they were very pleased with her. Most of the clients I have referred are African American. They differ in age, presenting concern, and socioeconomic background.

Camille A. Clay

After earning a bachelor's degree in psychology at Hampton Institute (now University), I completed a master degree in counseling psychology, then a two-year certificate in group and family therapy at the Psychiatric Institute of Washington, DC, and finally, a doctorate in counseling and human development from George Washington University. My dissertation topic was an analysis of the psychosocial development of middle-class African American adults. I have worked in adolescent, family, and community mental health in Washington, DC, and Bowie, Maryland. At Towson University, I was a senior counselor in the University Counseling Center and later assistant vice president for diversity. For the past 25 years, I have maintained a private counseling practice with adolescents, adults, couples, and families. I have been a full-time adjunct faculty and advisory board member for the graduate counseling program at University of the District of Columbia.

A long-time advocate for the counseling profession, I worked to establish licensure for professional counselors in the District of Columbia. I was the first person licensed there and hold license number 1. I served as chair of the D.C. Board of Professional Counseling from 1993 to 2004. A member of the American Counseling Association (ACA) and the American Mental Health Counseling Association (AMHCA), I serve on the Diagnostic and Statistical Manual (DSM-5) task force for both organizations. I also have been the North Atlantic regional director of AMHCA since 2009.

For me, counseling is creative enterprise which pulls together probably far more threads than I recognize at this point. Therapeutically and philosophically, I incorporate an integrative humanistic/existential approach. "Each of us craves perdurance, groundedness, community, and pattern; and yet, we must all face inevitable death, groundlessness, isolation, and meaninglessness" (Yalom, 1980, p. 485). Looking to the writings of Carl Rogers, I tend to be client-centered in that I allow the client to determine the direction and goals of our work together. The writings of Alfred Adler (2010), Rudolph Dreikurs (1967), and subsequent Adlerian thinkers have provided many useful tools and ways to frame what is occurring with my clients. I am also influenced by cognitive-behavioral therapies (CBT), initially in the work of Albert Ellis (2001) who trained and influenced the work of African American psychiatrist Maxie Maultsby* (the first African American psychology theorist I was aware of). Dr. Maultsby's writings always made sense to me for most of the people with whom I work. He developed rational-behavior therapy (RBT), which he saw as "an ideal cognitive behavioral therapy because it is comprehensive, short-term, cross-cultural, drug-free and produces long-term results" (p. 10). He wrote further,

> RBT is cross-cultural psychotherapy because it is acceptable to and effective for people whose ages, races, cultural values, and lifestyle preferences are widely different from those of their psychotherapists. . . . Hence, RBT is an excellent method for treating not only traditionally ideal psychotherapy candidates but also for treating people who are often neglected as psychotherapy candidates: adolescents, the elderly, the poor, and members of racial and ethnic minorities. (1990, p.10)

I regularly employ the tools and techniques of CBT, such as homework, thought stopping, reframing, and examining mistaken beliefs. Additionally, I use mindfulness techniques and hypnosis as needed. But more important, I think, than any tool or technique in the therapy process is the relationship that develops between client and therapist. The relationship is the primary curative factor. To be so, it must reflect an appreciation for the other; it sends the message that I (counselor) believe in you (client), that I value you as a human being, and that I will engage with you to help you change in the ways you choose (if I can). If I am not able to help you, then I will tell you so. My work with African Americans—males in particular—is often about undoing or lessening the effects of psychological damage. This is the damage that all too often ensues from being a Black man (or woman for that matter) in the United States. It may present itself in such problems as negative self-concept, low self-esteem, or an inability to trust or love. Even when my Black clients and I do not openly discuss race and racism, it is usually a consideration in my conceptualization of the case.

My work as a therapist is also influenced by my love of jazz. Jazz is said to be America's classical music. According to eminent jazz musicologist Billy Taylor*, "No other indigenous music reflects so clearly the American ideal of the individuals' right to personal freedom of expression. In many ways, jazz is a metaphor for the American idea of democracy." For me, jazz addresses Yalom's existential ultimate concerns of life—death, freedom, isolation, and meaninglessness. The four key elements of jazz—interpretation, improvisation, rhythm, and tempo—speak to the counseling process as well. I have always felt it necessary to interpret or translate the therapeutic idiom into one that connected with my clients. Each person, of course, is different from the next person so cookie-cutter approaches do not work. It is often necessary to improvise and to use all that I know to connect with my client. Charles Mingus*, a renowned jazz bassist, once said jazz musicians become composers when they improvise. Likewise, not only does each participant in the counseling session have his or her own rhythm and tempo but the counseling session itself has its own rhythm and tempo.

Betty Carter, my all-time favorite jazz singer, was said to have never sung the same song twice. She reinvented songs. She changed the rhythm and tempo each time. As she put it in a 1994 interview with writer Michael Bourne in the premier jazz magazine Downbeat, "I'm a jazz singer, there's no doubt about it. I reach and I take liberties. I do a lot of stuff—and it's mine. What you hear is me thinking at that time and the musicians behind me. They're reaching and growing at the same time." Jazz musicians often play past the notes and play what comes from the heart. In a jazz group, musicians play off each other. The lead soloist may set a tone then gives space for the others to support or amplify or perhaps take it in another direction. There is an apparent trust and appreciation for what each brings to the enterprise. They give each other space to develop and resolve musical ideas and questions and encourage their fellow players to go places they haven't been. They often embark on a musical journey not knowing where they will end.

Wynton Marsalis*, in the film *Jazz* by Ken Burns (2004), said, "The real power of jazz is that a group of people can come together and create improvised art and negotiate their agendas . . . and that negotiation is the art." I would paraphrase and relate the statement to therapy and suggest instead the following: the real power of therapy is that two or more people come together and create improvised art and negotiate their agendas and that negotiation is the healing.

In this case study I give the reader a sense of the client in his own words wherever possible.

The Case

Mr. Paul T is a handsome 59-year-old African American man. He is a natty dresser whose bearing and stride exude confidence. He smiles easily. A high-level public safety officer in a government agency, he supervises several people who are far better educated than he. He has taken advantage of all training and educational opportunities afforded him through his employment. A model employee for more than twenty years, he has advanced beyond his own expectations. Well regarded in his career and community, he is also a deacon in his church. He is married to a woman several years his junior and two children were born from this union. Presently, his children are adults who still live at home, a phenomenon not entirely uncommon in the United States. These adult children are called "millennials." A shorthand pop-culture way of describing the U.S. population born from 1980 to the present, millennials are youth whose lives are affected by a steadily declining U.S. economy, increased opportunities in education (especially across racial, ethnic boundaries as a result of the social movements of the prior three decades), and exposure to the rapid development of technology over the past four decades, which partly contributes to their desire for high living against a backdrop of an inflated housing industry in protected regions of urban areas (Pew Research Center, 2010).

Mr. T has three other children from a previous union that is described further below. Mr. T (as I always addressed him) sought counseling because he was experiencing marital distress and feelings of anxiety, guilt, and confusion. He did not want couples or marriage counseling because he and his wife had tried it before with limited success. This time he wanted to understand what was going on with him and in his words he wanted to "fix himself" before dealing with his marriage or family. He felt emotionally distant from his wife and children. He selected me from his health insurance provider list and assumed from the location of my office that I would be African American. In the United States, there are communities which can be described as mostly or overwhelmingly White, Black, or mixed (inferring an integration of people from different races). There are also "Chinatowns" and "Little Saigons," for example, which are usually low-income neighborhoods in large metropolitan U.S. areas that are composed mainly of Chinese and Vietnamese Americans, respectively, as well as other ethnic communities.

On the initial visit to my office, clients complete the Adult Checklist of Concerns (Zuckerman, 2008), the Patient Health Questionnaire 9 (PHQ 9), a nine-item depression screener developed by Kroenke, Spitzer, & Williams (2001), and the Generalized Anxiety Disorder Assessment (GAD-7) (Spitzer, Kroenke, Williams, & Lowe, 2006), a seven-item anxiety questionnaire, adult version. In addition, they complete forms providing basic identifying information. Clients complete the GAD-7 and PHQ-9 at the beginning of each subsequent visit to allow me to track shifts in depression and anxiety symptoms over time. On the initial visit Mr. T checked no symptoms on the GAD-7 form. On the PHQ-9 he indicated, at intake, that for several days he had little interest or pleasure in doing things; that he was feeling down, depressed, or hopeless; and that he was feeling bad about himself or that he had let himself or his family down. On his checklist he indicated childhood issues, health and medical concerns, marital concerns, housework and chores, sharing duties, oversensitivity to rejection, self-centeredness, and sexual issues. The concerns he most wanted help with were self-centeredness and marital distance.

I've found that providing an atmosphere that is professional yet comfortable is very important for African American clients, particularly men. I strive to make the space and everything about the service communicate to clients, "You are welcome," "You are valued," and "You are respected." I have a friendly, usually smiling receptionist as well as a front office that has a rather formal front desk, a few chairs, colorful art work, and plants. There is a sizable candy box where the offering changes weekly but likely includes bite-sized chocolates, chewy sours, Tootsie rolls, and so on— usually candy to which everyone from teens to seniors can relate (targeting candy classics, I often hear from my senior visitors statements like "Oh, Squirrel Nut Zippers! They were my favorite" or from twenty-somethings "Do you have any Smarties?"). In addition to candy, we offer bottled water to each visitor. In the counseling room, rattan and wood loveseat and chairs are covered with comfortable pillows. The furniture, pillows, artwork, book cases filled with books, and soft light from lamps convey openness, warmth, comfort, and safety. I intentionally try to create or establish a healing environment.

The Context

The United States of America is composed of 50 states, the District of Columbia, and the territories of American Samoa, the Federated States of Micronesia, Guam, North Marianas, Puerto Rico, and the Virgin Islands. Before its establishment as a nation, this land was home to an indigenous population which Italian explorer Christopher Columbus labeled "Indians" because he believed he had landed in India. The population of American Indians or Native Americans has dwindled precipitously since Columbus' pillage (Takaki, 1993; Zinn, 2010).

With a population of over 312,000,000 (U. S. Census, 2010), it is also the world's third most populous country. Located mainly on the North American continent, it is considered the most ethnically diverse nation in the world. It has been labeled the "land of opportunity" for immigrants from countries throughout the world, a setting where generations of immigrants have established themselves economically, socially, and politically and continue to do so. The United States also is considered around the world as a "superpower," a phrase coined by a geostrategist named Nicholas Spykman (1944) to refer to the country that has considerable influence over a global hegemony. This influence is political and economic in scope, to be sure, but also includes military, cultural, geographic, and demographic influences. Although Spykman named other countries as superpowers at the time of his writing—specifically the Soviet Union and the British Empire, there is controversy over which countries constitute current superpowers and even if *any* superpower today exists (Bacevich, 2011).

The influence of the United States over all parts of the world has taken on both positive and negative connotations. For example, as one of the wealthiest nations in the world, the United States has and continues to provide aid to countries in need when there are natural disasters like the tsunami in Indonesia or the earthquake in Haiti and Chile, and these funds that come from the United States are derived at the government level, from nongovernmental organizations, and from private donations by private citizens. The American government has provided assistance to countries during human-made catastrophes as well as in the case of mass killings and intractable wars. Americans travel abroad extensively for leisure, business, and humanitarian reasons. In terms of negative influence, the United States has contributed to and started wars based on an interest in resources within other countries and its political allegiance with different factions within countries. Although the U.S. government has provided substantial monetary help to other countries to help them build economies, notably through the Marshall Plan, there are steep criticisms regarding the reasons for these allegiances and how, in cases where the humanitarian need is great, there has been no or little outpouring of monies or military force (Lewis, 1993; Zinn, 2010). The United States has participated in several wars, beginning with a revolution that culminated in its independence from the Kingdom of Great Britain in 1776 to the current war in Afghanistan. The United States' wealth is seated in multinational corporations and individuals. Indeed, although 49% of the country is considered middle class, a group toward which politicians aspire to curry favor during election times, there is a distribution of wealth in which 84% of the wealth in the country resides with the rich and super rich who constitute one percent of the population (e.g., Chang, 2011). This contingent also controls much of the media and, therefore, is able to wield influence over the messages and images that are conveyed both domestically and abroad. This condition of extreme inequality is not always perceived by citizens in United States (see Winslow, 2011), owing in part to a lack of disclosure about the financial dealings that occur in the country and, as alluded to earlier, owing to a media conglomerate that projects notions of the country's greatness as accessible to anyone. The popular stories of author Horatio Algers invoke the notion that any individual who wants to achieve is capable of doing so, and thus, tends to downplay class exploitation and entrenched, unresolved oppression on the basis of race and gender. Other U.S. problems include a proliferating culture of materialism which influences psychological well-being (see Kasser & Kanner, 2003) against a backdrop of increasing poverty among Americans.

There clearly is a mixture of sentiments concerning the U.S. government's actions both domestically and abroad, freedom of speech, the extent of opportunities for vocation and avocation, and the ideals that form the U.S. Constitution as the bedrock of further progress—the building blocks of optimism for a country for which many people continue to have hope. Still, deep injustices occur within the nation on the basis of race, gender, and socioeconomic status. In regards to the juxtaposition of race and class which are highly intertwined, thousands of authors from a spectrum of disciplines and throughout the different eras of U.S. history have eloquently penned narratives (e.g., Baldwin*, 1962; Ellison*, 1952; Jacobs, 1970; Muhammad, 2010) and scholarly analyses that describe how the phenomenon of race, a derivative of structural racism, has shaped and continues to shape interpersonal relationships, both between and within different racial groups. Attention to the phenomenon reached a pitch on the world level following World War II, epitomized by the emergence of the U.S. Civil Rights

Movement. Visual displays and reports of Whites' harsh treatment toward Black Americans were documented in media and spread more pervasively than in the past. Although space does not allow for a thorough examination of the history of deeply entrenched racism in American sociopolitical landscape, readers are urged to read from an enormous range of books on the topic, a few of which are cited here: I. Wilkerson's (2011) *The Warmth of Other Suns*, R. Takaki's (1993) *A Different Mirror*, and J. H. Franklin* and A. Moss's* (2000) *From Slavery to Freedom*.

Mr. T is a Black American who is likely the descendant of the estimated 10 to 15 million people who were shipped from Africa during the Atlantic slave trade between 1450 and 1860 (Franklin* & Moss*, 2000). African Americans comprise about 13.5% of the U.S. population and approximately 54% of them live in the southern region of the country. The history of the experiences of African-descended people in the United States is a lengthy and complicated one; we point specifically here to the psychological impacts of Blacks in this chapter. One of the impacts is that Black Americans experience conflicting messages about the society and ultimately about themselves. The famous W. E. B. Du Bois* (2005), a founder of the National Association for the Advancement of Colored People (NAACP), refers to this conflicting experience as the "warring souls" of Black people, on one hand being culturally American and feeling a desire to be part of the mainstream and, on the other, knowing that they can never be part of the mainstream because of the hostility and hatred that they are barraged with. Furthermore, Du Bois and other theorists point to the relevance of African cultural traditions that have served African Americans through the generations and which are often resisted because of the negative images projected in society of Africans specifically and African-descended people in general. Fanon* (1967), a Martiniquean psychiatrist who wrote about the need for a liberation of Black people throughout the world, pointed out that psychological theories crafted by Whites have generally ignored the impacts of oppression on psychological development and functioning— not only for African-descended people but also for Whites and everyone ostensibly affected by it. The emergence of a Black or African American psychology over the past five decades has been one response to the lacunae in traditional psychology training programs of theories that are inclusive of Black people's experience and in some cases, inclusive of African traditions (Jones*, 1991; Neville, Tynes, & Utsey*, 2009).

The Africanist presence in the United States has had an undeniable impact on the American landscape, from the origins of the first uniquely American art forms like vaudeville, rhythm and blues (which later morphed into rock and roll), and jazz to current political debates about immigration, health care, school reform, and urbanization, which are threaded with needed discussions over the role of race and racism. However, the persistent diminishment of the humanity of non-White people and simultaneous inflation of

Whites as relatively superior in worth (with Whites, like other racial groups, being identified as a function of social constructions; see Bonilla-Silva, 2009) continues to pervade virtually all aspects of American life.

These macro-systems problems ostensibly influence individuals. Mr. T is an African-American man who is mature in age and has achieved certain commonly held successes in his life—a committed relationship, children, prestige, and a steady income. Yet, he feels incapable of expressing love and feels detached and isolated from his wife and children as well as remorse for his distancing behaviors. In assessing the needs of Mr. T, it is not merely to determine *if* race or culture plays a role in reaching an understanding of him. It is to *know* that race and culture as well as his socialization as a man who has experienced abuse and isolation as a child are crucial to any practitioner who takes seriously the role of Mr. T's need for healing. The therapist needs to probe freely, naturally into the myriad aspects of Mr. T's life. Because racism is a phenomenon that is often misunderstood to refer narrowly to acts of discrimination and even dismissed altogether, it is the onus of the practitioner to resist or overcome conformity to U.S. societal norms by achieving sound knowledge about racism. It is also the onus of the practitioner to determine how racism's impacts influence the lives of clients—any client. When the phenomenon is understood as one that entails issues of power, dominance, and as a cultural invention that is woven into the fabric of American society, then practitioners are better capable of making assessments, developing authentic relationships, and attending to their clients than when they conform to society's minimization of it. To understand the complexities of racism is also to understand the self and one's relationships with others irrespective of racial and other boundaries (see Thompson and Alfred, 2009). African Americans may seek counseling with African American professionals because there can be an unspoken understanding of racism's presence and potentially less tension within these unions than in those when the practitioner is not Black.

Psychological History of the Client

I, Camille Clay, conducted a modified-lifestyle assessment (an Adlerian structured interview technique including the family constellation and early recollections) to glean his early childhood views of how he saw himself, the world, and others in it. He was the oldest of four children–each a year apart. In his descriptions of family members, he had very little to say about his mother; however, he spent time talking about his father who was not only the disciplinarian and provider but also his abuser. Mr. T's father ruled the household. As he stated, "whatever he said went." Mr. T was close to his siblings, often taking up for them in the neighborhood and when there were conflicts in the family. He remembered a close relationship with his maternal grandmother with whom he spent a lot of time.

"She loved me," he remembered with a smile. His main memories, however, were that his father verbally and physically abused him constantly. He never felt he belonged in the family. He thought, "I'm getting these beatings for nothing." He was beaten more than his siblings, but they, too, did not escape punishment. One day he and his sister were watching Elvis Presley on television when the sister said she thought Elvis was "so cute." Her father knocked her across the room saying, "Don't you ever let me hear you say a White man is cute!" Then he straddled our client and said, "And don't you ever bring a White girl in here." According to Mr. T, his father hated White people. Whenever he approached his mother for help, she would not intercede. She would tell him he should obey his father. Mr. T thought his mother believed her husband to be a good provider who was good to her and merely stern with the children.

When he was 12 years old, he moved from the U.S. Midwest to Washington, DC, where he found that not only did he not fit in with the family but also that he did not fit in with the neighborhood. His Midwest accent was seen as "talking proper" and he did not dress in appropriate "DC style." He was harassed and bullied by the local teens. As he put it, he became a bad kid real quick. He fought almost every other day. A slender boy, he used sticks, rocks, or whatever he could to best his adversaries. He was "a menace to society" and his father continued to punish him at will. He also never wanted to believe that the man he was told was his father was really his father, often wondering, "How could he be my father and treat me this way?" On one occasion when he was 16, he went back to visit his grandmother in his Midwestern hometown. At a family gathering, a family friend greeted young Mr. T and said, "I just saw your father." Confused, he asked if the woman had been in DC and from there it was revealed that his real father lived in that town and that most family members and townspeople knew about his biological father. He asked her for his father's address and met his biological father that day. His father said he had not been in contact with him because his mother had asked the father not to contact her or Mr. T. From then on, he maintained a relationship with his biological father, unbeknownst either to his mother or stepfather. He stayed in touch and visited whenever he could. But importantly, Mr. T was relieved to know that the man he thought to be his father, who had treated him so badly, and for whom he could do nothing to please, in fact was not his biological father.

But well before the age of 16 he had already concluded that he was unloved and unlovable (or would have if it were not for his grandmother). He was not accepted surely; and the world was a mean, unpredictable, and unsafe place. Mr. T could not trust his parents to protect him and therefore his fighting and other rebellious behavior was justified. Even though he was a smart student, he rebelled against a life that was mean and unfair, and at age 16 he left school and entered the Job Corps to prepare to enter a trade. (The Job Corps is a federal program that began in 1964 under the presidential administration of Lyndon B. Johnson as part of his War on Poverty agenda. It serves youth from ages 16 through 24, providing free educational and job training services.) After completing the Job Corps program, Mr. T worked various odd jobs but nothing that provided the income he wanted. He worked when he could but was also involved in street life. He became involved with a young woman and had three children with her. At the age of 23, Mr. T joined the military. Being in the military was difficult for him since following rules and dealing with authority had not been his strong suit. Using his combination of street sense and intellectual ability, he was able to get through four years of military duty and was subsequently honorably discharged. One of his earliest accomplishments was to sit for the high school equivalency exam. Rather than taking the preparation course, he asked to take the test first. Permitted to do so, he passed the test with ease. For the most part, his work in the military was in administrative settings.

Mr. T joined the military because he needed an income he could count on for his family. Although he regularly sent funds for his children, his partner felt she had been abandoned. She sent several "Dear John" letters ending the relationship when he was overseas. By the time he returned home, she was involved with another man. In a period that extended from early adolescence until after his military career was completed at the age of 27, he was constantly in fights, he abused drugs and alcohol, and he repeatedly had close encounters with law enforcement. Because he was in the street so much and because she had moved on, he was never there for that family. It was not long after his discharge that he met and married a woman 11 years his junior and had two more children.

With his new wife, he continued working at one job then another and continued his drug involvement as well. They lived with her parents, who encouraged them to attend their church. At one point they became *saved*, that is, they joined the church and gave their lives to God. Actually it was a joke to them. They even toasted and drank alcohol in celebration. About that time, the crack epidemic hit DC and he told of being caught up in it. He used and sold crack cocaine. Eventually he moved out, left his family, and moved in with the drug dealers. He was driven each day to his drug-selling post where he worked until he was picked up and he was given as much crack as he wanted for his personal use. It was all a haze; he said, he supposes he was having a good time until one morning he got up, pulled up and fastened his pants, and they fell to the floor. He couldn't believe he had lost that much weight. He described falling to his knees crying and asking God to help him get out of there and return to his family. He made a bargain with God that if He allowed him to get out of the situation of drug abuse and illegal activity, he would join the church and serve Him for the rest of his life. He told his housemates he was leaving, fully expecting them to block his exit. To his dismay, the housemates allowed him to leave. Then he called his wife and told her he wanted to come home. She said he could if he agreed to get into a drug treatment program. Although he agreed, he initially was placed on waiting lists as the need for drug rehabilitation in the city was so great. He tried 12-step programs but was never able to find a program that was the right fit for him. He felt God had told him he needed to be prayed for to seal his commitment to change his life. According to Mr. T, once he received that prayer he never looked back. Later, he and his wife joined and seriously committed their lives to the church. From that point forward, he kept his word and worked to provide a better life for his family. He found low-paying jobs at first but then finally qualified for an entry-level government job. He continued to advance step-by-step until he was at the top of that career ladder. By the time he came back to his wife and family, Mrs. T. had been taking care of the children with the financial and moral support of her parents. She had become accustomed to managing her life and the lives of the children socially and financially without him. And because of what they had been through, it took a long time for her to believe that this turnaround was real. In addition, they disagreed on childrearing. He reported that his wife spoiled the children and that his wife felt that he, in contrast, was overly strict. In many ways, he felt they were her children and because he was tired of fighting about them, he left the child rearing to her. This arrangement went on for several years, so even though Mr. T's situation at work was progressing quite well, his home life with his wife and children was characteristically detached, lonely, and profoundly unfulfilling.

The Treatment

We met at least twice a month for almost five months. Mr. T talked about his family of origin and about his fears and failures as husband and father. Initially the focus of the sessions was Mr. T, then as he began feeling better about himself, the therapy turned next to his relationship with his children and finally, to his relationship with his wife. From the beginning, Mr. T welcomed the opportunity to tell his story and to try to make sense of it. Often fighting back tears, he remembered a painful past. He often expressed amazement that he survived through such turbulence in his life.

The First Phase of Treatment

In the first few weeks of initial homework exercises (see following examples), history taking, and relationship building, Mr. T gave me a picture of how he saw himself, the world, and others in it. As reported previously, he told me what he saw as his main problems and he told me how to help him. That he shared so easily told me he felt comfortable, listened to, and valued in that setting. His responses (in italics) on two early homework assignments outlined the work to be done. Also revealed in these responses are Mr. T's suggestions on how he wanted me to help him.

1.   What do you need and deserve by virtue of the fact you're a member of the human race?

Physically—*I deserve to be treated like I treat others. I need to be able to be myself. I have the basic right to make my own decisions. I deserve to make life as pleasant as I possibly can. I need to make my family happy.*

Emotionally—*I need to be stroked positively and reassured that I can do whatever I put my mind to. I need to be loved by my family. I need to be more loving and caring. I need to communicate in a more positive manner.*

2.   What keeps you from doing that which is necessary to get your needs met?

Being withdrawn and stubborn; not caring how others around me feel, being out of touch with reality.

3.   What are your clues that your needs are not being met or that someone is taking advantage of you?

Physical Sensations—*The feeling that I can't make my family happy, being tired, and not wanting to participate in family things.*

Thoughts—*I want so bad to change the way I'm living life right now; I feel life is too short to be feeling the way I do.*

Feelings—*Sometimes sad, sometimes in love, sometimes happy but nothing consistent but low times.*

For another exercise entitled Selfish or Self-Sufficient he wrote the following:

1.   Name 5 things you do to take care of self.

Practice good hygiene; take my medication; wear clothes that make me feel good; go to a counselor to get help.

2.   Taking care of myself is . . .

Doing things that will keep me healthy and mentally sound and feeling good about myself.

Being selfish is . . .

doing things that I want to do no matter what anybody says or feels about what I'm doing as long as I please my own desires.

3. If you don't take care of yourself, who does?

In most cases no one.

4. What has stopped you from taking care of yourself in the past?

Depression, not feeling loved or cared for.

In subsequent sessions, Mr. T added to these written prompts. He rather eloquently and clearly told me he was depressed. He grew up with the perception that he was an outsider; he was angry and rebellious. The world was a mean and unsafe place. People couldn't be trusted for the most part. They will hurt you if you give them a chance. He fought, at first literally, and later figuratively, to be included and accepted in his family and in the community. With a determination to survive, he essentially turned his life around and became successful in his chosen field. His work life helped lessen some of the emptiness and feelings of worthlessness he experienced. But inevitably, these efforts were not enough, especially as he was surrounded by people who needed him to love them and to be someone who was grounded in a love for himself.

Shortly after his first visit, Mr. T was diagnosed with diabetes. Until then he had relatively few health problems. Then he was confronted with questions about what this meant, how he needed to change his life style, and his dietary habits. What did this mean in terms of his view of himself, about mood changes, and about his sex drive? He felt once again he was in this alone. It is noteworthy here that African Americans are twice as likely to be diagnosed with diabetes as non-Hispanic Whites. In addition, they are more likely to suffer complications from diabetes, such as end-stage renal disease and lower extremity amputations. The 2007 age-adjusted death rate from diabetes was 42.8 per 100,000 persons for Blacks, more than double the rate for Whites (19.8) (Centers for Disease Control Office of Minority Health and Health Equity, n.d.). Clark*, Anderson*, Clark, and Williams* (1999) address the role of racism and the stress that arises from it in the health problems of Blacks in general.

Mr. T's health status, age, and the problems in his marriage combined quite likely prompted a life review. In terms of what he wanted out of the therapy from me, Mr. T. told me he wanted to be respectfully listened to, heard, and challenged. He wanted to tell his story, to "put it all out there" in an atmosphere of acceptance, and he wanted help understanding and making sense of it. Additional goals for our work together were to examine his negative beliefs and distorted thinking patterns and challenge and change them. He also wanted to forgive himself and those who had mistreated him. Although he was a Christian and embraced the concept of forgiveness, he realized that he held onto his pain and shame and had not forgiven his mother for keeping from him the identity of his real father and for not protecting him from his stepfather. He also found it very difficult to forgive his stepfather for years of abuse and himself for not being the husband and father he thought he should be. A large part of Mr. T's treatment was to guide him in challenging the irrational beliefs that prompted him to feel depressed about his life circumstances. What was raised continually in each session was followed by the exercises which not only helped the client to focus on new thoughts and practice the cognitive restructuring techniques, but also to think more repetitively about his worth as a person, father, and husband. There were several strengths I used to reinforce Mr. T's acuity at achieving more rational thinking. For example, Mr. T realized many years ago that the abuse he experienced was senseless and that neither he nor his siblings deserved it. The constant attention and affection of his grandmother served as a powerful inoculation of beliefs that could very well have become more deeply set. Moreover, Mr. T knew after taking the GED that he had the cognitive ability to do well academically. He had to acknowledge at some point that he held back and kept himself from realizing the power within him to beat the odds of living a destructive lifestyle. He also held on to a faith in God and kept to his promise to continue his praise toward God as he made efforts to leave the destructiveness behind. Knowing that he was successful and well-regarded at work was not enough to keep his soul assured. He somehow knew that this compartmentalized lifestyle was not a life he wanted to live. As difficult as it was for him to face certain truths, such as the neglect of his partners and children, he showed a drive to endure the difficulty.

Mr. T and His Children

For his children, Mr. T was to the extent he could be, a good provider financially. However, he felt incompetent as a father. Two of his three children from his first marriage were lost to the streets and the third, the oldest who is female, refused to have anything to do with him. From this first marriage, one son was killed in a street fight, the other was imprisoned for life for killing a man. In both cases, he became involved with the children after these tragedies occurred. He tried, unsuccessfully, to learn the circumstances around his son's death. He supported the other son through his trial and sentencing. His son from his current marriage was recently released from jail for drug possession. His guilt related to his sons was palpable: "I should have been there. I should have been a better father." Although Mr. T dealt with some of this guilt through his faith, he continued to bombard himself with his negative self-talk.

Mr. T began to examine some of his negative self-talk, "I cannot possibly be a good father," and replace it with realistic statements like, "I *can* learn how to be the father I want to be." He was able to see how ill prepared he was for the roles of loving father and husband. His only real model of fatherhood was his stepfather. He was able to connect his desire for a loving father with the fact that he was not being one for his children. Like his stepfather, he took care of his family financially but was not there emotionally for them. I challenged his belief that he could not become a better, more loving father by reminding him what he learned to do in his work life in spite of the fact that he was a high school dropout and helping him realize this was another learning opportunity. We talked about how he had inadvertently passed down the pain inflicted by his stepfather and that this intergenerational pattern may continue with his grandchildren unless he consciously worked to turn it around as he had done in other areas of his life.

His children did not know his personal story. He had never shared with the children with whom he lived the history he shared with me. I thought his son might benefit from knowing the adversity his father had overcome and could use that model as the son tried to rebuild his life after prison. As we continued, I encouraged him to take a more active role with his daughter. On one occasion, he took the daughter who was unemployed to a job fair and demonstrated for her how to talk to potential employers and then supported her while she tried new behaviors. He believed this outing proved to be successful because they shared the experience rather than him lecturing or telling her what she should do. On another occasion, he invited his daughter for an afternoon in the park where he told her about aspects of his history (I suggested he tell only as much as he felt comfortable with). He was pleased to find that she was receptive and used the opportunity to share with him information about her life. Other homework involved doing things with his family members or having specific conversations with them. I suggested, at times, he operate as a participant observer in these situations allowing him to maintain some distance but not doing so without being active (taking note of certain dynamics, for example). Mr. T heeded this suggestion which helped him ease into new roles and helped move him closer to his family. I listened to and supported his views about family members at times and other times confronted or challenged the mistaken beliefs which led to his pain. I call it "spitting and stroking." Dreikurs (1967) talked about spitting in a client's soup by stating that the client may continue to drink it but it would not taste the same. The term stroking relates to another Adlerian concept of encouragement. As a therapist or a jazz musician, I did what I did, gave him space, and watched where he took it. In the context of a developing relationship, combined with exploration of feelings, an opportunity to tell his story of his past and negotiate how much was enough to reveal and for me to probe, Mr. T was able in time to reframe what he saw as his tragic childhood into the triumph it was.

Mr. T and His Wife

Mr. T loved his wife and admired her strength and talents. At the same time, he had particular difficulties with her being demanding and controlling him and everyone around her. He understood that much of this related to that time when he was an irresponsible partner, but he had long since shown that he was no longer that guy. He and his wife had loud arguments at times, but more often, he was indirectly aggressive. For example, he would come home from work at the end of the day and sit in his comfortable chair in the living room in front of the TV and not move to help with the household responsibilities. He allowed her to take over the children, the household funds, and much of the decision making, and he quietly resented her for it. He often refused to engage with the family. Her major complaint was that he was selfish. He agreed but believed since childhood he had to take care of himself because no one else would. Again, he had no basis for a loving, trusting relationship. In the sessions, he often vented about disagreements they had. After a rant, I'd ask, "And what did you do?" He'd acknowledge what he was doing was ineffective. It didn't get him what he wanted. Then I'd invite him to think through with me other ways of handling the situations. Sometimes he'd try other approaches, sometimes with success, others not.

During some of the final sessions of treatment, I invited Mrs. T to the sessions, but these proved very difficult. It was clear that this aspect of Mr. T's needs would require more time and more willingness on both his and his wife's parts to let go of some long-held resentments they had of one another in relation to the marriage.

Evaluation of the Treatment

After about four months, Mr. T reported feeling better. At about this time point, Mr. T indicated no depression symptoms on the PHQ-9 that he completed at the beginning of each visit. He reported getting along better with his children. He said when he first came to counseling, he felt like a failure; he was congested and filled-up with painful thoughts and feelings. He explained that he felt free to express his feelings during counseling, whereas at home when he expressed his thoughts and feelings it lead to an argument. In counseling he was able to "download so much stuff" and subsequently, he was able to show more respect and appreciation for his family following these sessions. He said that his wife recognized changes in his behavior as well. She could see that he was taking time for and being more attentive to her and to the children and that he stopped bickering. As he put it, "She could see it was working."

Although I would have liked for him to continue a little longer than he wanted, I saw the counseling experience with Mr. T as successful because he expressed that he felt it was. In addition, by the end of the sessions he was better able to make connections about past and present; he openly acknowledged feelings in ways he could not before and he was able to challenge negative beliefs, for example, that he was unloved and unlovable and that he could not be a loving father and husband and change negative feelings and behavior.

I think that all clients tell us how to help them if only we, as therapists, are capable, willing, perceptive, and open to hearing them. Mr. T gave me an added gift in that he wrote instructions in the first exercise: "I deserve to be treated like I treat others," "to be able to be myself," "to be stroked positively and reassured that I can do whatever I put my mind to." He told me, "In most cases no one cares," and what stopped him from taking care of himself in the past was "not feeling loved and cared for." And so I provided a respectful, caring atmosphere in which I gave him space to be himself, to tell his story, to hear himself telling his story, to see and hear me reacting to his story, and to help him deconstruct his story, and to make sense of it. I allowed him to be the lead soloist and I played behind him to start and as that continued he began to feel more comfortable and secure and to take risks exploring feelings and trying new behaviors. I constantly reassured him that he could do whatever he put his mind to. That I am an African American woman in his age group and from DC may have helped us form a mutually respectful relationship, but I think more important is the fact that I listened with acceptance and without judgment. My stance with clients generally is not to know their stories but to communicate a willingness to learn about them from them, whether they are from the other side of town or the other side of the world; regardless of age, circumstance, religion, or lack thereof. I believe that this stance, in part, is how I am able to build trusting relationships with them.

Conclusion

At first glance, Mr. T appeared to be a Black man who had overcome the damage of institutional racism, one who lived the American Dream—married, two children, gainfully employed—in fact, he worked his way up from entry level to very near the top of his career ladder and was a leader in his church and in his community. On the surface, he even appeared happy. But as he talked, he revealed the scars of the damage were very much there, and they were very well hidden. He entered counseling because he was suffering. In spite of his success, he was unhappy in his marriage and had been recently diagnosed with a disease he would have to manage for the rest of his life. Within the context of a supportive, safe counseling relationship, Mr. T was able to sift through the wreckage of his turbulent past. He was able to come to terms with his parents' failures and those of his own. He had faith in God to help motivate him to live, what African-centered theorist Linda James Myers (1988) calls an *optimal* life in which he recognizes himself to be the manifestation of a higher being. He, therefore, is called to do more, be more, and become true to himself. Telling his story with someone who understood the context (could vibe with his rhythm and tempo), who did not judge him, and who continuously encouraged him, freed him to express his feelings, to think new thoughts, and try new behaviors (to improvise and play variations on his themes and patterns). While we don't know why his father was angry at White people or why his mother would sit by and allow her husband to mistreat her children for what seemed to be solely material reasons, Mr. T lived through what it is like to experience the parenting of two people whose *suboptimal* lives (see Myers, 1988) likely were influenced by racism and poverty. Both probably thought they were raising their children to survive in a difficult and dangerous world. Mr. T was fortunate to be exposed to a grandmother whose life may not have been any less encumbered by racism, but who celebrated his humanity by loving him. "She loved me," he said touchingly.

Mr. T could very well have continued on for the rest of his life with the more damaging legacy. But to do so would mean self-pitying (Why me?) or wanton aggression toward others (I'm going to hurt people just as much as I was hurt). We are elated that Mr. T chose to heal in a constructive manner. His healing entailed extending himself to his family as he was able to see the linkages between his experiences and those of his children. He began to understand why he was, as his wife labeled him, being emotionally distant from his family. He began to change how he thought and felt about himself and his family. And he felt good about himself and the work he did. At his advanced age, he merely took on new lessons to add to his repertoire. In the future, these lessons may find him deepening his relationships with his wife and family and tapping further into his love of self, others, and God.

References

Adler, A. (2010). *Understanding human nature*. Eastford, CT: Martino Fine. (Original work published 1927)

Althen, G., & Bennett, J. (2011). *American ways: A cultural guide to the United States*. Boston, MA: Nicholas Brealey.

Bacevich, A. (2011, November 13). *The Era of US dominance is coming to a close*. *Global Policy Forum*. Retrieved from http://www.globalpolicy.org/component/content/article/152-challenges/50993-the-era-of-us-dominance-is-coming-to-a-close.html

Baldwin, J. (1962). *The fire next time*. New York, NY: Vintage.

Bell, D. A. (2008). *Race, racism, and American law*. New York, NY: Aspen.

Bonilla-Silva, E. (2009). *Racism without racists: Color-blind racism and the persistence of racial inequality in America*. Lanham, MD: Rowman & Littlefield.

Bourne, M. (1994, December). Betty Carter: It's not about teaching. It's about doing. *Down Beat, 61*, 17.

Burns, K., & Novick, L. (Producers), & Burns, K. (Director). (2004). *Jazz: A film by Ken Burns*. [Motion picture]. United States: Florentine Films and WETA TV.

Carter, R. T. (2007). Racism and emotional injury: Recognizing and assessing race-based traumatic stress. *The Counseling Psychologist, 35,* 13–105.

Centers for Disease Control (CDC) Office of Minority Health and Health Equity. (n.d.). *Office of Minority Health and Health Equity (OMHHE)*. Retrieved from http://www.cdc.gov/minorityhealth/

Cesaire, A. (2001). *Discourse on colonialism*. New York, NY: Monthly Review. (Original work published in 1955).

Chang, H-Y. (2011). *23 things they don't tell you about capitalism*. London, UK: Brownsbury.

Clark, R., Anderson, N. B., Clark, V. R., & Williams, D. (1999). Racism as a stressor for African Americans: A biopsychosocial model. *American Psychologist, 54,* 805–816.

Dreikurs, R. (1967). *Psychodynamics, psychotherapy and counseling*. Chicago, IL: Alfred Adler Institute.

Du Bois, W. E. B. (2005). *The souls of black folk*. New York, NY: Simon & Schuster. (Original work published 1903)

Ellis, A. (2001). *Overcoming destructive beliefs, feelings and behaviors*. New York, NY: Prometheus.

Ellison, R. (1952). *The invisible man*. New York, NY: Vintage.

Fanon, F. (1967). *Black skin white masks: The experience of a black man in a white world*. New York, NY: Grove.

Franklin, J. H., & Moss, A. A. (2000). *From slavery to freedom: A history of African Americans*. New York, NY: Knopf.

Hilliard, A. G. (1997). *SBA: The reawakening of the African mind*. Gainesville, FL: Marare.

Jacobs, H. (1970). *Incidents in the life of a slave girl, written by herself*. Boston, MA: Bedford/St. Martin. (Original work published 1861).

Jones, R. L. (1991). *Black psychology* (3rd Ed.). Berkeley, CA: Cobb & Henry.

Kasser,T., & Kanner, A. D. (2003). *Psychology and consumer culture: The struggle for a good life in a materialistic world*. Washington, DC: American Psychological Association.

Kelley, R. D. G., & Lewis, E. (2005). *To make our world anew I: A history of African Americans to 1880*. Cambridge, MA: Oxford University.

Kroenke, K., Spitzer, R. L., & Williams, J. B. (2001). The PHQ-9: Validity of a brief depression severity measure. *Journal of General Internal Medicine, 16,* 606–613.

Lewis, D. L. (1993). *W. E. B. Du Bois: Biography of a race, 1868–1919*. New York, NY: Henry Holt.

Maultsby, M. C. (1990). *Rational behavior therapy*. Appleton, WI: Rational Self Help Books.

Muhammad, K. (2010). *The condemnation of blackness: Race, crime, and the making of modern urban America.* Cambridge, MA: Harvard University.

Myers, L. J. (1988). *Understanding the Afrocentric worldview: Introduction to an optimal psychology.* Dubuque, IA: Kendall Hunt.

Neville, H. A., Tynes, B. M., & Utsey, S. O. (2009). *Handbook of African American psychology.* Thousand Oaks, CA: Sage.

Parham, T. A. (2009). Foundations for an African American Psychology. In H. A. Neville, B. M. Tynes, & S. O. Utsey (Eds.). *Handbook of African American psychology* (pp. 3–18). Thousand Oaks, CA: Sage.

Pew Research Center (February, 2010). Millennials: Confident, connected, open to Change. Retrieved from http://pewsocialtrends.org/files/2010/10/millennials -confident-connected-open-to-change.pdf

Pieterse, A. L., & Carter, R. T. (2007). An examination of the relationship between general life stress, racism-related stress, and psychological health among Black men. *Journal of Counseling Psychology, 54,* 101–109.

Robinson, R. (2001). *The debt: What America owes to Blacks.* New York, NY: Plume.

Spitzer, R. L., Kroenke, K., Williams, J. B. W., & Lowe, B. (2006). A brief measure for assessing generalized anxiety disorder: The GAD-7. *Archives of Internal Medicine, 166,* 1092–1097.

Spykman, N. (1944). *The geography of the peace.* New York, NY: Harcourt, Brace and Company.

Takaki, R. (1993). *A different mirror: A history of multicultural America.* Boston, MA: Back Bay.

Thompson, C. E., & Alfred, D. M. (2009). Black liberation psychology and practice. In H. A. Neville, B. M. Tynes, & S. O. Utsey (Eds.). *Handbook of African American psychology.* Thousand Oaks, CA: Sage.

Thompson, C. E., & Carter, R. E. (1997). *Racial identity theory: Applications to individual, group, and organizational interventions.* Mahwah, NJ: Lawrence Erlbaum.

United States Census Bureau. (2010). *2010 Census.* Retrieved from http://2010 .census.gov/2010census/

U. S. Department of Health and Human Services, The Office of Minority Health. (n.d.). *African American profile.* Retrieved from http://minorityhealth.hhs.gov/ templates/browse.aspx?lvl=2&lvlID=51

Utsey, S. O., Bolden, M. A., & Brown, A. L. (2001). Visions of revolution from the spirit of Frantz Fanon: A psychology of liberation for counseling African Americans confronting societal racism and oppression. In J. G. Ponterotto, J. M. Casas, L. A. Suzuki, & C. M. Alexander (Eds.). *Handbook of multicultural counseling* (2nd edition, pp. 311–336). Thousand Oaks, CA: Sage.

Watts, R. J., Williams, N. C., & Jagers, R. J. (2003). Sociopolitical development. *Journal of Community Psychology, 31,* 185–194.

West, C. (2001). *Race matters.* Boston, MA: Beacon.

White, J. L., & Parham, T. A. (1990). *The psychology of Blacks: An African American perspective* (2nd Ed.). Upper Saddle River, NJ: Prentice Hall.

Wilkerson, I. (2011). *The warmth of other suns: The epic story of America's great migration.* New York, NY: Vintage.

Winslow, L. (Executive Producer). (2011, August 11). Home of the brave, land of the poor. *PBS News Hour.* Washington, DC: MacNeil/Lehrer Productions. Retrieved from http://www.pbs.org/newshour/bb/business/july-dec11/making sense_08-16.html

Yalom, I. D. (1980). *Existential psychotherapy* New York, NY: Basic Books.

Zinn, H. (2010). *A people's history of the United States.* New York, NY: Harper Perennial Modern Classics.

Zuckerman, E. L. (2008). *The paper office: Forms, guidelines, and resources to make your practice work ethically, legally, and profitably* (4th Ed.). New York, NY: Guilford.

Working With a Chinese Immigrant With Severe Mental Illness

An Integrative Approach of Cognitive-Behavioral Therapy and Multicultural Case Conceptualization

Munyi Shea
Frederick T. L. Leong

Introduction of the Authors

"How will (participants') acculturation levels influence the focus and delivery of your intervention?" The first author, Dr. Munyi Shea, was once asked this question about a research project she conducted with Asian immigrant youth. Several years later, the second author confronted her with a similar question, pertaining to a clinical context involving Asian immigrants. Both authors sensed the growing interest in integrating current psychotherapy models with a culturally responsive approach. Nevertheless, they found the literature on service delivery to Asian clients—especially to those with severe mental illnesses—lacking (Hwang, 2007; Hwang, Miranda, & Chung, 2007). Dr. Frederick Leong's question led to a discussion about how contextual factors could be consistently integrated in therapists' treatment formulation and how within-group, differences such as acculturation levels could be explored and explicitly addressed in the

clinical process. Since then, the two authors have collaborated to examine these subjects (see Shea, Yang, & Leong, 2010).

Dr. Munyi Shea is a counseling psychologist and currently a faculty member in the Department of Psychology at California State University, Los Angeles. She was born to ethnically Chinese parents and raised in Hong Kong and mainland China. She attended college as an international student in the United States and received her doctorate in counseling psychology from Teachers College, Columbia University. Her primary clinical training was in community mental health, working with individuals and families of diverse ethnic-cultural backgrounds and often low-income status. Her migration experience and professional training have significantly impacted her worldview and endeavors.

Dr. Frederick Leong is a leading scholar in multicultural psychology. He is a professor in the Department of Psychology at Michigan State University in both the Clinical and Organizational Psychology programs. He is also director of their Consortium for Multicultural Psychology Research. Having been trained in psychodynamic psychotherapy at the University of Maryland and Dartmouth-Hitchcock Medical Center, he has been involved in training graduate students in both psychodynamic and cross-cultural psychotherapy for the last 25 years. In 2008, he was invited to give a state-of-the-art lecture on his Cultural Accommodation Model of Psychotherapy (Leong & Lee, 2006) at the World Congress of Psychotherapy in Beijing.

The Practitioner

Dr. Shea

During my undergraduate orientation, a counselor spoke about potential challenges associated with cultural adjustment. At that time, these "potential challenges" did not worry me; my primary goal as an international student in the United States was to succeed in my academic studies. (I did not even realize until later that this orientation was separate from the one offered to U.S. nationals.) Jazzed by the variety of courses and the endless possibilities of social adventure, I felt well prepared to tackle any challenges. Over time, my contact with the mainstream culture intensified. Yet, I found it increasingly challenging to fully embrace the culture, or to be fully embraced by it. This realization was puzzling, paradoxical, and inconsistent with my learning experience. How could it be that over time I was becoming more accustomed, more assimilated to the dominant group, but felt more alienated? How could it be that I was becoming more fluent in the language but still stumbled in relationships and social processes? Simultaneously, I was slipping away from my culture of origin—its language, values, traditions, and customs. The experience of constantly navigating and negotiating both cultures was frustrating. The realization that I no longer had a strong footing in either culture was scary and painful.

The bewilderment, burdens, and tensions of operating across cultures cannot be easily resolved; however, they can be overcome. In my confusion and conflicts, I reached out to my friends, family, and mentors; found solace in reading and spirituality; and began a journey of seeking and authoring meaning. All these endeavors helped me reconnect with my work and my community and made me feel more grounded. The journey also steered me further in my quest for meaning and ultimately to studies in counseling psychology.

My graduate program emphasized multicultural psychology and a postmodernist perspective, both of which challenge the notion of "objective truth," including the definitions of psychological "normality" and "abnormality." Both perspectives advocate a collaborative stance between the therapist and the client: as the therapist takes a "not-knowing" or curious position, he or she becomes more attuned to the diversity of clients' voices and appreciates clients' subjective realities. Although I was clinically trained in the mainstream theoretical orientations and therapy models, such as psychodynamic therapy and cognitive-behavioral therapy (CBT), I attempt to integrate my academic background and philosophies with my clinical work. The training in psychodynamic and CBT approaches has given me a breadth and depth of knowledge, strategies, and techniques to apply during the treatment process. The multicultural and postmodernist perspectives challenge me to consider my position and relation to my clients and how my clients and I construct the meaning of therapy together. I have learned to allow room for clients to tell their stories so I can understand problems and challenges from their perspectives. Rather than merely applying diagnostic labels and implementing treatment without cultural accommodation, I believe that it is important to understand the deeper meaning of clients' psychological problems, distress, functioning (whether adaptive or maladaptive), and indigenous coping within their sociocultural contexts.

Theoretical Framework for Our Case

The theoretical framework that guides our conceptualization and discussion of this case is the cultural accommodation model (CAM) (Leong & Lee, 2006). The movement toward identifying and delivering evidence-based treatment or empirically supported therapies has gained footing in the field of psychology over the last two decades. Evidence-based practice or empirically supported therapies refer to those treatment modalities that have been demonstrated to be effective and superior to another treatment or a placebo during randomized controlled trials in experimental settings (Chambless & Hollon, 1998). Although research on the efficacy and effectiveness of empirically supported therapies (EST) and empirically validated therapies (EVT) for racial and ethnic minority groups remains limited (Chambless et al., 1996), scholars in multiculturalism have argued that psychologists should not ignore or dismiss scientific evidence when conducting cross-cultural psychotherapy. Psychologists instead should examine the potential benefits of the mainstream (Western) psychotherapy model beyond the dominant racial-cultural group (i.e., White Americans in this case), while simultaneously attending to culturally specific elements of the mainstream model that may not be applicable to other racial-cultural groups (Leong & Lee, 2006).

To bridge the gap in applying mainstream theoretical models and implementing evidence-based treatment in culturally diverse groups, Leong and Lee (2006) proposed the CAM. This model provides a theoretically sound guide for conducting effective and culturally responsive therapy with racial-ethnic minority groups. The CAM process involves two major steps that are briefly summarized here: the first step seeks to identify and acknowledge cultural gaps and limitations of mainstream psychotherapy models with racial-ethnic minorities; the second step involves identifying constructs and variables that are culturally specific to the ethnic minority group (e.g., cultural values and beliefs, immigration experiences) and that need to be incorporated in the mainstream model and psychotherapy process. Further, the authors suggested that the process of identifying and accommodating culture-specific constructs and variables should be informed by current literature and scientific studies with racial-ethnic minorities; for instance, studies on acculturation, racism, and cultural values.

Against this backdrop, the authors of this chapter explore a case of a Chinese immigrant from Vietnam with prominent mood and psychotic symptoms, using an integrated approach of a mainstream, evidence-based treatment—cognitive-behavioral therapy—and a culturally responsive clinical perspective—multicultural case conceptualization. We demonstrate that cognitive-behavioral therapy can be an effective treatment approach with a Chinese immigrant with severe and persistent mental illness. Further, we describe how the client's contextual conditions and racial-cultural factors are taken into account when we formulate the treatment goals and intervention. The discussion focuses on a three-month clinical process during which Mr. P. was seen by Dr. Munyi Shea in a partial hospital program in the United States.

The Case

At the time of his referral to a partial hospital program, Mr. P. was a 47-year-old, single, heterosexual, Chinese American man from Vietnam, who lived in a group home and attended a rehabilitation day-treatment program. Mr. P. had been discharged from the psychiatric unit at a general hospital. Prior to his psychiatric admission, the group home staff had expressed concern that Mr. P.'s symptoms had worsened. These symptoms included increased agitation, arguments with staff over rule infringement and medication regimen, and bizarre behaviors such as "chanting" and "dancing." He had—on one occasion—expressed suicidal thoughts: "Buddha tells me to kill myself."

Mr. P.'s primary language is Cantonese (a Chinese dialect); he speaks little English. Interview and therapy sessions were conducted with Dr. Shea (referred to in this chapter as *the therapist*) in his primary language. During the intake interview, Mr. P. was pleasant and cooperative. His speech and behavior were within the normal range. He did not display a dysphoric sad mood, nor did he appear elated. Occasionally he would giggle—an affect that appeared to be incongruent with the contents of the interview. He told the therapist that the "voices" in his head made him laugh. These voices were of his mother and friends, who told him to "study hard." However, Mr. P. was amenable to the therapist's redirection and able to focus throughout the interview. Mr. P.'s chief complaint at that time was "My nerves are all messed up. My thinking is confused." He could not elaborate what he was confused about, but stated that he suffered from a chronic headache. Mr. P. showed some insight into his conditions: He reported that the precipitating events leading to his recent hospitalization had been his "singing" and "dancing," which bothered other residents in the group home. But he stressed that there was no aggressive intent on his part. When asked about his suicidal ideation, Mr. P. adamantly denied it, saying, "I believe in Buddhism, and we are told to be good. We cannot hurt others or ourselves."

Personal History

Mr. P. was born and raised in an ethnically Chinese family in Ho Chi Minh City, formerly known as Saigon, Vietnam. He was the middle child of five children with one older brother, one older sister, and two younger sisters. Both of his parents were agricultural workers. Mr. P. described his father as "distant," and his mother as "warm" and "caring." He had a conflictual relationship with his older siblings; he recalled being physically abused by his older brother and verbally abused by his older sister. Mr. P. appeared fearful and reluctant to talk about his older siblings; he did not wish to elaborate on the abuses. According to Mr. P., there was no major medical or psychiatric history in his family.

Although his family struggled intensely with poverty and discrimination by the Vietnamese, Mr. P. did not report any other remarkable experiences during his childhood years. He attended Chinese-speaking elementary and middle schools until age 14 and then decided to drop out and find work. Mr. P. appeared proud of the fact that all his schooling was in Chinese and noted to the therapist, "I don't know or speak Vietnamese very well." After trying several odd jobs, he became involved in a smuggling business.

In the early 1980s, Mr. P. (then a teenager) and some friends fled Vietnam's new Communist regime in search of safety. He paid a "snake-head" (a person or a gang that is involved in human smuggling) to traffic him via boat to Hong Kong. Mr. P. remarked that his parents were ailing and his older siblings were married with children. "It would be too expensive to pay for the entire family to go." The rest of the family remained in Vietnam. They were later expelled to a southern province in China.

Clinical History

Mr. P. was first hospitalized in the early 1980s in Hong Kong. During this time, Mr. P. was under a great deal of stress arising from political, social, and economic situations. After arriving in Hong Kong from Vietnam, he was admitted to a refugee camp. To pass time and make money, Mr. P. started working "under the table" in several restaurants and factories. He reported drinking a lot of coffee and sleeping very little in order to work long hours. Over time, his supervisors and friends noted that he became increasingly irritable, incoherent, and uncooperative. Eventually, Mr. P. was taken by his friends to a local psychiatric hospital. There, he was diagnosed with bipolar disorder. Mr. P. did not seem to understand the diagnosis. As he said, "I just thought I had a lot of energy, and I needed to work a lot [to make money]. I did not sleep, and I collapsed. That is it."

Shortly after his discharge, Mr. P., along with other Vietnamese refugees, was admitted to the United States under the Humanitarian Operation. He settled in an urban city in the Northeast. Since then, he has had close to 20 psychiatric admissions due to recurrent manic and psychotic episodes. These are characterized by symptoms of persistently elevated mood, increased irritability, auditory hallucination, grandiose and control delusions, hyperactivity, and a substantially decreased need for sleep. Owning to his chronic mental health condition and limited English proficiency, he has not held steady jobs in the United States since his immigration. Mr. P. relies on government subsidies as his major source of income.

Mr. P. had been diagnosed with bipolar disorder and schizoaffective disorder by various therapists. Prior to the time discussed here, he had been receiving approximately once-a-month psychiatric care from a Cantonese-speaking outpatient psychiatrist in a general hospital, who described Mr. P.'s condition as "persistent" and "grim" in spite of continued anti-psychotic medication treatment. "He believes he is powerful and able to communicate with people through extraterrestrial systems," the psychiatrist told the therapist. Mr. P. briefly saw a Cantonese-speaking social worker but terminated that therapy for unknown reasons. Additionally, Mr. P. had been referred to a rehabilitation program that consisted of primarily Vietnamese immigrants. According to Mr. P., he left the program because of "language and cultural mismatch." Mr. P. was a smoker, but he had no history of substance abuse or significant medical problems.

The Context

Considerable research has shown that the schizophrenia spectrum of mental illness is associated with genetic factors (Tsuang, Stone, & Faraone, 1999) and neurobiological vulnerabilities, such as alterations in brain structure (Belger & Dichter, 2006), an excess of the neurotransmitter dopamine, and dopamine's interaction with other neurotransmitters (Kapur & Lecrubier, 2003). Nevertheless, many researchers have suggested the significant role of environmental, psychological, and social factors; in particular, the effect of life stressors on the developmental trajectory of schizophrenia (Phillips, Francey, Edwards, & McMurray, 2007). In Mr. P.'s case, there were tremendous experiences in his history that embodied his identity as an immigrant and a refugee and multiple sociocultural factors that potentially instigated and became interwoven with the expression of his severe mental illness. In the following, we examine a few salient factors in Mr. P.'s migration and acculturative contexts that likely affected his psychological health and were important to consider in his treatment conceptualization and planning.

Migration History and Context

Mr. P. was born in Saigon in 1960 during the Vietnam War. Although he was unable to elaborate this part of his personal history, he alluded to disliking an environment that was combative and highly conflictual—one that was exemplified by his own family dynamics as well as the larger political climate. Mr. P. was a teenager when Saigon fell, and at that time, he became increasingly worried about the brutal rule of the new Communist government and the discrimination against ethnic Chinese. His fear of being persecuted or sent to a reeducation camp, coupled with a bleak future for job opportunities, led him to flee Vietnam to Hong Kong.

According to Mr. P., the refugee camp in Hong Kong was filthy; fights (verbal and physical) were frequent. He abhorred these tensions and rejected any association with the people there; instead, he sought solace in his Buddhist faith and focused on seeking jobs. One of the highlights Mr. P. recalled of this short stay was his ability to maintain several part-time jobs in restaurants and factories. Nonetheless, Mr. P. was constantly worried about being arrested for working illegally and deported back to Vietnam. "I worked a lot . . . to make a lot of money quick. I felt happy when I was working." Unfortunately, this abundance of energy, drive to succeed, elated mood, and unusual optimism signaled an impending manic episode, which eventually led to his first psychiatric hospitalization.

Acculturation Context

The term *acculturative stress* is used to describe the feeling of tension and anxiety caused by the demands of a new environment on a person to adapt and change (Berry & Kim, 1988). Like many new immigrants (Rhee, 2009), Mr. P. struggled with economic hardship and significant acculturative stress associated with changes on individual (e.g., language spoken), structural (e.g., social network), and sociocultural (e.g., customs and norms) levels. Despite his high hopes for greater freedom and better job opportunities in the United States, Mr. P. was quickly plunged into an environment that was unfamiliar and challenging. At first, he tried to establish his footing by doing menial jobs (e.g., washing dishes in a restaurant) and making new friends. However, Mr. P.'s low educational level and limited English-language proficiency not only limited his vocational choices but also circumscribed his social network. Although he attended free English classes offered in the community, his ability to concentrate and retain information was impaired by his mental condition. Further, his life was punctuated by the chronicity and persistence of his mental illness. Mr. P. never quite returned to his premorbid level of functioning. Consequently, he could not maintain employment. Unable to make a living and care for himself, Mr. P. began to receive government subsidy and live in a group home.

After his multiple hospitalizations for mood and psychotic episodes, Mr. P.'s social network collapsed. Friends, especially those with families and children, became distant. He lived in a group home comprised predominantly of Whites and African Americans, with whom Mr. P. was cordial but had little in common. Although Mr. P. had been referred to ethnic specific rehabilitation centers, including a day treatment program with Cantonese-speaking social workers, he did not follow through and eventually terminated the service due to a long commute. Mr. P.'s experiences illustrate the paucity of culturally appropriate assessment and mental health services and the logistical challenges in delivering them (Sue & Sue, 2007). They also speak to a profound sense of sadness, loss, and resignation among recent immigrants as a result of social alienation and cultural marginalization.

The immigration process also brought upheaval and disruption to Mr. P.'s emotional support systems. Mr. P. was separated from his family for an extended period of time before he returned to China to visit them. During that visit, he learned that his father had passed away and his siblings had established their own lives in different towns. Mr. P. related to the therapist that he missed his mother but did not feel close to his siblings. That was his last and only visit to see his family.

Several studies have shown that stressful premigratory experiences can lead to severe mental health problems among Vietnamese immigrants or refugees, including elevated rates of depression, posttraumatic stress disorder (PTSD), and panic disorder (Abueg & Chun, 1996; Hinton et al., 2001; Kinzie et al., 1990; Tran, 1993). Postmigratory stressors such as language barrier, low socioeconomic status, disruption of family integration, and social isolation can exacerbate acculturative stress and increase the risk for mental health symptoms (Rhee, 2009; Shea, Yang, & Leong, 2010; Shen & Takeuchi, 2001). Mr. P.'s early exposure to war trauma and his experience of living in highly unsettled and alienated environments may have resulted in his constant feelings of trepidation and uncontrollability and a lens tinted with distrust. All these factors affect the way he sees and interacts with the world (i.e., cognitive schemas), as well as his psychological experiences and symptom manifestation (discussed in the next section).

Other Racial Cultural Factors

Culture not only shapes immigrants' psychological experiences, but also orchestrates the expression of their psychological distress, such as *somatization*. As research has suggested, Asians and Asian Americans tend to express their distress and emotions through somatic metaphors (Cheung, 1995; Hwang, 2007; Shea et al., 2010) and emphasize somatic symptoms over psychological difficulties in assessment and treatment (Yang & Wonpat-Borja, 2006). When Mr. P. first arrived at the unit, he did not endorse any mood symptoms but complained about his perennial headache. This became a starting point of his work with the therapist.

Religious and spiritual beliefs also inform a client's worldview, conception of mental health, and coping mechanisms. Scholars and practitioners generally view religious and spiritual faith as a protective factor against psychological distress (Sanchez & Gaw, 2007) and a source of resilience and coping among Asian immigrants (Inman, Yeh, Madan-Bahel, & Nath, 2007). It is imperative to attend to the interaction of religious and cultural contexts. For instance, committing suicide is not explicitly forbidden by Buddhism and Hinduism (Leong, Leach, Yeh, & Chou 2007). However, the act of killing oneself may be regarded as selfish and disruptive to interpersonal harmony; hence, it is deplored in the Asian cultural context.

Beyond cultural factors, scholars have posited that race is a central organizing principle for our society as well as for our clinical work (Hardy & Laszloffy, 2008). It is not only important for therapists to recognize racial-ethnic differences but also important to understand differential meanings and values we attach to these differences. For instance, Mr. P., at one point, was referred by the inpatient clinicians (who are primarily White) to a rehabilitation day program that mainly served Vietnamese Americans following his discharge from an inpatient unit. He appeared particularly upset about this arrangement and said to the therapist, "I don't even speak Vietnamese." The misunderstanding and the misplacement should not simply be attributed to language barriers or carelessness. The confusion about Mr. P.'s ethnic background, cultural practice, and language preference might reflect clinicians' biases and assumptions of those who are racial-culturally different as well as their privileges of choosing not to see or understand group differences. Thus, it is critical for therapists to examine their daily operation as a racial-cultural being and its powerful implications for their interventions and interactions with clients (Constantine, Miville, Kindaichi, & Owens, 2010). In this case, the clinicians needed to learn to grasp the complexity of

Mr. P.'s sociocultural realities, become aware of widely varied within-group ethnic, linguistic, religious and cultural differences, and challenge their stereotypic views about racial-ethnic minority groups (Constantine et al., 2010; Hardy & Laszloffy, 2008; Sue & Sue, 2008).

Therapist's Role and Stature Relative to Mr. P.

The therapist was born outside the United States and shared with Mr. P. a similar ethnic background and the same spoken dialect. Nevertheless, her migration and acculturation experience was very different from Mr. P.'s. She first came to the United States as a student with financial and cultural resources. Unlike Mr. P., she never had to struggle with safety or survival issues, nor did she flee her home country and leave her family behind out of fear for her own life. She was accepted by her communities in the United States, and did not need to worry about where she would live and whom she could befriend because of stigma. She received advanced education that broadened her horizon of career opportunities and afforded her upward mobility and social class privileges in the dominant culture. Yet in some ways, she could relate to Mr. P., feeling at times the excruciating pain of being far from family and emotional support systems; challenged or misunderstood because of values, beliefs, and practices; or perceived as a perpetual foreigner.

These similarities and differences prompted the therapist to examine Mr. P.'s operation as an ethnic minority in the dominant culture as well as her own. Their shared language facilitated dialogue and contributed to a better understanding of Mr. P.'s distress and challenges. Yet the differences in their age, gender, social class, and life experiences reminded the therapist to be mindful of her values and assumptions of normality and privileges; to be humble and listen to Mr. P.'s story; and to explore meaning from his perspective, not hers.

The Treatment

Treatment Goals and Planning

When Mr. P. first arrived at the unit, he presented active delusions and hallucinations without prominent mood symptoms. He told the therapist and psychiatrist that his father was "Chairman Mao"; and, his mother, "Queen Elizabeth II." He also believed that he had the ability to maintain world peace by manipulating his thoughts. Additionally, he reported hearing voices—mostly his mother's voice telling him to "learn English" and "study hard." Mr. P. did not present significant negative symptoms.

Upon reviewing Mr. P.'s psychiatric history and course, the clinical team generally supported a diagnosis of schizoaffective disorder. There was a period of time when Mr. P.'s psychotic symptoms persisted without the presence of mood symptoms. The key intervention recommended by the psychiatrist was medication. Mr. P. was treated with a combination of Depakote (Valproic acid), Lamictal (Lamotrigine), Clozaril (Clozapine), and Abilify (Aripiprazole) for his manic and psychotic symptoms. He was also prescribed Tylenol for his chronic headache and Ativan for his anxiety and instructed to take them as needed.

In addition to pharmacotherapy, CBT and multicultural case conceptualization (MCC) approaches were included in Mr. P.'s treatment plan. CBT (Beck, 1976) emphasizes helping clients examine maladaptive thought processes and recognize underlying cognitive schemas that trigger erroneous automatic thoughts and generate negative behavioral and emotional responses. Treatment often centers on modifying clients' faulty thinking patterns by substituting more realistic appraisals and enabling them to learn adaptive behavioral responses. Although it was once suggested that symptoms of schizophrenia would not respond to any form of individual therapy, recent treatment research has demonstrated that CBT can be an efficacious treatment for schizophrenia (see review by Turkington, Kingdon, & Weiden, 2006).

The MCC approach, on the other hand, focuses on mental health practitioners' ability to identify and integrate salient racial-cultural issues into their case conceptualizations of etiology and treatment formulation (Ladany, Inman, Constantine, & Hofheinez, 1997). Instead of attributing a client's symptoms and illness trajectory to a simple biological cause (e.g., imbalance of neurotransmitters) or psychosocial cause (e.g., homelessness, limited family support), this approach prompts therapists to engage in a closer examination of the sociopolitical and cultural contexts—such as race, ethnicity, gender, social class, and religion—that shape a client's identity, developmental experiences, and storytelling. Furthermore, MCC goes beyond understanding the intrapersonal factors on the client's part and stresses the importance of considering the practitioner's covert biases and assumptions in clinical assessment and diagnosis. MCC also emphasizes the racial-cultural dynamics between client and practitioner as well as the interpersonal processes within the treatment milieu (Constantine et al., 2010; Shea et al., 2010).

It has been suggested that MCC can augment mainstream theoretical orientations (e.g., psychodynamic, CBT, rational-emotive behavioral therapy, humanistic, and family systems) to promote comprehensive case conceptualizations and culturally responsive service delivery (Constantine et al., 2010). In Mr. P.'s case, the MCC approach fits well with the premises of CBT. First, both CBT and MCC promote client-practitioner collaboration, which generates shared formulations of problems through guided discovery (Kingdon & Turkington, 2005). Second, both methods value clients' subjective experiences. One of the central tenets of CBT for schizophrenia is to respect and understand the personal meaning of clients' experiences (Sullivan, 1962)—including their beliefs, feelings, and behaviors—without directly challenging the reality basis of their experiences or colluding with their delusions (Turkington et al., 2006). Similarly, MCC encourages viewing clients' symptoms in the larger context and being interested in the specific narratives based on their racial and ethnic experiences. These strategies underemphasize preconceived ideas of normality and abnormality, help uncover culturally oriented conceptions and expressions of mental health problems, reduce Eurocentric biases in assessment and diagnosis, and facilitate understanding of how cognitions and behaviors may be adaptive from clients' perspectives (Constantine et al., 2010).

Informed by the CBT and MCC perspectives, the therapist took a collaborative stance in developing treatment goals with Mr. P. The first and foremost problem Mr. P. complained about was his chronic headache. He also stated that he would like to return to the English-speaking vocational-based rehabilitation center that he had previously attended. Prior to his recent hospitalization, Mr. P. had attended that center regularly and was engaged in some simple cleaning tasks.

Although it might seem that treating Mr. P.'s positive psychotic symptoms would be the paramount goal, it soon became clear to the therapist that his delusions and hallucinations were not particularly distressing to him or harmful to others. What piqued the curiosity of the therapist were the perseverative, ritualized, and almost soothing qualities in Mr. P.'s narratives of his delusional thoughts and voices, which led the therapist to explore the protective function of these symptom manifestations and their effect on Mr. P.'s mood.

The additional concern was Mr. P.'s history of erratic behaviors as described in consultation and liaison meetings. Specifically, group home staff members were troubled by Mr. P.'s "irritability" and "argumentative attitude." There were also the instances of "chanting" and "dancing," which he claimed were part of his religious rituals. Furthermore, therapists and staff at the partial hospital program noted that Mr. P. was "encroaching interpersonal boundaries" with some of the other clients. Mr. P. did not seem to agree with others' assessment of his behavior, insisting that he had no ill intention toward staff or other clients. Despite the dispute, Mr. P. agreed that it would be helpful to discuss different social norms and expectations that govern interpersonal processes to reduce misunderstanding between him and others.

After some discussion, the client and therapist generated three treatment goals: (1) understand Mr. P.'s positive symptoms and explore the effect on his mood and daily functioning, (2) enhance his interpersonal effectiveness, and 3) develop an integrative care plan that would address his physical and mental health concerns and promote his quality of life.

Course of Treatment

This section presents a brief summary of the work between Mr. P. and the therapist, which occurred during three months of meeting twice to three times a week, for 30 to 45 minutes each time. The initial-estimated length of Mr. P.'s intervention was six to twelve weeks. The purpose of the partial hospital treatment is to provide transitional support and clinical care for clients who no longer need the intensive inpatient treatment, but who would benefit from more structured and frequent therapeutic encounters before they are discharged to outpatient facilities.

In the first few sessions, Mr. P. claimed that he was confused in his new surroundings and did not understand why he was attending the partial hospital day treatment program. In one moment he would repeatedly urge the therapist to let him "go home," and in the next, he would say to himself, "I need to study . . . I need to learn English." The initial sessions focused on developing empathy, respect, and unconditional positive regard for the client as well as fostering trust and honesty (Turkington et al., 2006). The therapist acknowledged Mr. P.'s confusion and encouraged him to discuss how the partial hospital program could be helpful and to explore what a home meant to him.

Within a week, Mr. P. felt more situated and became comfortable sharing his histories. Despite bitter complaints about his headache, Mr. P. began minimizing this problem and was reluctant to address it. He said, "I have been telling my doctors about my headache for almost thirty years, and they can do nothing about it. I just take Tylenol." The therapist, hoping to better understand Mr. P.'s vulnerabilities as well as stressors that trigger his headache, used *Yang Sheng* ("nourish life")—a Chinese concept related to cultivating a lifestyle that promotes inner balance and longevity—to stir Mr. P.'s interest in a dialogue about his health. Mr. P. became engaged and stated that Buddhism also encourages its believers to maintain physical health. These dialogues about inner balance and longevity seemed to help Mr. P. gain a new perspective on his health concerns and reduce the intensity of his headache symptoms.

Working with his attending psychiatrist, the therapist suggested that Mr. P. keep a log of his daily routines and dietary patterns, while simultaneously arranging a medical appointment for Mr. P. to undergo further examination. When Mr. P. returned with his log and observations, two vices appeared to be especially relevant to Mr. P.'s symptom of a headache: heavy smoking and caffeine consumption. He drank coffee continually throughout the day, which led to restlessness, difficulty falling and staying asleep at night, and chronic fatigue. Although the medical test revealed no organic causes for his headache, quite soon after the adjustments of his dietary habits (including increased hydration and decreased caffeine intake), Mr. P. appeared more physically comfortable. He reported improved sleep quality, higher levels of energy, and less frequent headache symptoms. Nevertheless, Mr. P. refused to give up smoking.

The therapist also noted that the onset of Mr. P.'s chronic headache coincided with a very stressful period of his life: living in the refugee camp in Hong Kong. Moreover, Mr. P. at times in therapy complained about headaches when he was confused or anxious: "My nerves are all messed up. They hurt my brain." These complaints made the therapist mindful of how Mr. P. might express his emotional and psychological pain through somatic metaphors. The therapist then directed the session toward understanding Mr. P.'s fear and anxiety rather than reverting to simple medication intervention.

Mr. P.'s delusional thinking revolved around bizarre and grandiose themes, but he did not display systematic, elaborate, or well-organized delusions. He tended to focus on a few specific themes and talk about them in a ritualized manner. As stated earlier, he believed that his father was "Chairman Mao," his mother was "Elizabeth Queen II," and he could maintain world peace and stop the Iraq War by concentrating on his thoughts. (He could not elaborate what thoughts these were.) Mr. P. also appeared to experience persistent auditory hallucination. Mr. P. would often start giggling in the middle of the therapy and say, "It's my voices . . . so funny. My friends are talking to me now." Once during group therapy, he leaned toward the therapist and lowered his voice. "Can you hear that? The air conditioner is sending me messages, telling me to be good and to keep this group in peace. Now! Now! Hear it!"

Mr. P.'s delusions were refutable. There were multiple times when he clearly identified that his parents were agricultural workers in Vietnam, and his account of family and migration history was rather consistent. The therapist used a CBT technique known as "inference chaining" to examine personalized meaning underneath Mr. P.'s delusions (Kingdon & Turkington, 2005). An example follows:

Mr. P.:   "I can control world peace. I just need to concentrate."

Therapist: "Could you please tell me what controlling world peace means to you?"

Mr. P.:   "When I concentrate, the world will be safe. Everyone will be happy."

Therapist: "So it is important to you that the world is safe and everyone is happy. Could you please tell me why it is important?"

Mr. P.:   "Yes. When it is not safe and people are unhappy, people argue."

Therapist: "Can you give me an example of a time when you felt that the world was not safe?"

Mr. P.:   "Like when I was in the refugee camp in Hong Kong; people fight and argue all the time . . ."

Dialogue like this opened a well of revelations. In a sense, the delusion was bypassed and instead channeled to explore important feelings and experiences in Mr. P.'s life. He subsequently related to the therapist how life had been challenging and chaotic for him as a refugee and immigrant. Even though Mr. P. had never verbally endorsed any feelings of loneliness or sadness, his responses at times suggested that he longed for connections and safety. For instance, when asked about what "Chairman Mao" and "Queen Elizabeth" would do for him if they were really his parents, Mr. P. sank into his deep thoughts; his eyes became moist. "I miss my mother," he said.

The details of Mr. P.'s hallucinations were explored to identify situations that increased the likelihood of his experiencing the sensation of hearing and becoming troubled by voices. It appeared that Mr. P. was most likely to hear voices when he was in a group setting or during an intense conversation that generated uneasiness or anxiety. The voices were mostly associated with familiar people: his mother and his friends, who encouraged him to study, learn English, and excel in the United States. They seemed to have a soothing effect. Instead of trying to convince Mr. P. that his auditory hallucination was a marker of schizophrenia, the therapist focused on uncovering stress factors that could exacerbate his symptom of anxiety and on enhancing his coping skills. For instance, the therapist suggested that Mr. P. excuse himself from the (therapy) room and go get a cup of water when he felt overstimulated. Mr. P. was also encouraged to keep to a regular routine of exercise, diet, and sleep that would help reduce stress.

Throughout his stay in the program, Mr. P. was cordial and made attempts to socialize with other clients. However, several therapists and staff expressed discomfort with Mr. P.'s insistence on shaking their hands every day and his habit of giving away cigarettes to other clients. Mr. P. argued, "I am just treating them like my brothers and sisters." The therapist and Mr. P. engaged in a constructive discussion about varying sociocultural norms and expectations for interpersonal boundaries and relationships in his country of origin and the United States as well as alternative ways of socializing besides offering cigarettes and smoking together. Mr. P. was quick to respond to the feedback and replaced handshakes with a simple wave and greeting; this change demonstrated Mr. P.'s ability to reason and to adapt to the demands of reality.

Evaluation of the Treatment

About eight weeks into the partial hospital treatment, Mr. P. was making steady progress and his condition was much improved and stabilized. Mr. P.'s physical and psychological symptoms had significantly reduced. His mood was stable, his affect was congruent, and his behaviors were appropriate. More importantly, he was engaged in the treatment and had not missed any individual or group therapy sessions.

As the clinical team began to discuss Mr. P.'s discharge plan, Mr. P. had a disagreement with a nurse about his medication regimen. During the incident, he became angry and agitated, yelled and cursed at the nurse, and left the unit. When Mr. P. later returned, he was calmer but claimed that he was still irritated by the nurse's attitudes. Since irritability was one of the main concerns expressed by Mr. P.'s care workers and an emotional state that might underlie his suicidal thinking, Mr. P. and the therapist completed a functional analysis of this outburst. Functional analysis is a technique frequently used in behavioral therapy to understand factors that contribute to the development and maintenance of a behavior. Mr. P. was asked to identify (1) situations or emotions that triggered his outburst and (2) the pros and cons of his behavioral consequences. Both the therapist and Mr. P. were made aware that his outbursts were often triggered by specific emotional states and interpersonal exchanges. For instance, disagreements with people—especially authority figures—reminded him of prior physical and verbal abuse by his siblings, which then triggered feelings of fear, anxiety, and anger. Mr. P. equated the nurse with his sister and said, "Just like my older sister, [she is] so controlling." The therapist and Mr. P. then explored alternative explanations for the nurse's seemingly controlling behaviors. Mr. P. was able to better understand the nurse's intentions. Nevertheless, Mr. P. still felt disabled in his communication with people around him, as if he would not be heard or understood even if he screamed. After making an assessment based on the CAM, it struck the therapist that this profound sense of not being understood underlies Mr. P.'s struggle with loneliness and loss as an immigrant with severe mental illness. He remains alienated from the mainstream society due to linguistic and cultural difficulties and marginalized by his own ethnic cultural group due to the stigma attached to mental health problems.

It became clear to the therapist that she would need to be more proactive—not only as Mr. P.'s therapist but also as a cultural broker and advocate when formulating Mr. P.'s discharge plan. She began to contact community leaders and other bilingual therapists in the area and consulted with several community agencies and hospitals to discuss Mr. P.'s discharge plan and appropriate outpatient care. In addition to medication intervention from his psychiatrist, Mr. P. would receive continued care from a bilingual outpatient clinical team. A Cantonese-speaking case worker would visit Mr. P. in his group home on a weekly basis and act as a liaison, while a clinical social worker would conduct therapy. Furthermore, the therapist, together with the case worker, met with Mr. P.'s group home staff to discuss pertinent issues such as rule negotiations (e.g., religious rituals, medication regimen), diet, exercise, and financial management. The therapist also collaborated with the clinical social worker in that they would both provide treatment to Mr. P. during a 2-week period prior to his discharge. The parallel treatment aimed to provide a smooth transition for Mr. P. and an opportunity to address any potential issues.

Mr. P.'s input was also sought during the discharge planning. He specifically requested to go back to the vocational-based rehabilitation center where he could work. Instead of seeing his request as a futile attempt or a wild dream by an immigrant who had failed to succeed in the mainstream society, the therapist saw hope and resilience.

Conclusion

In this chapter, we illustrate how to integrate a mainstream, evidence-based treatment—cognitive behavioral therapy—with a culturally sensitive approach in case conceptualizations and interventions. Consistent with the CAM of psychotherapy (Leong & Lee, 2006), we believe that cultural factors can serve as major moderators of both the process and outcome of psychotherapy and need to be accommodated in order to provide culturally appropriate and responsive interventions. We hope this discussion will inspire therapists and trainees to (1) engage in a dialogue with colleagues and clients to understand how clinical discourse is intertwined with a client's personal narrative as a racial-cultural being; (2) uncover embedded sociocultural factors that may influence a client's idioms of distress, symptom manifestation, and coping strategies; (3) examine their own cultural imperatives, biases, and assumptions as well as resources and assets that can be powerful tools to shape case formulation and treatment course; and (4) become more proactive in their advocacy for infusing racial and cultural factors in clinical assessment, treatment planning, delivery of services, and practicum class and supervision discourse. As our society becomes increasingly diverse, we must challenge our conception of the traditional therapist's role in order to understand the broader context of our clients' experience, integrate social justice in our practice, and seek knowledge and collaborations from our local, national, and global communities.

References

Abueg, F. R., & Chun, K. M. (1996). Traumatization stress among Asians and Asian Americans. In A. Marsella, M. Friedman, E. T. Gerrity, R. M. Scurfield, & M. Raymond. (Eds.), *Ethnocultural aspects of posttraumatic stress disorder: Issues, research, and clinical applications* (pp. 285–299). Washington, DC: American Psychological Association.

Beck, A. T. (1976). *Cognitive therapy and the emotional disorders.* New York, NY: Harper & Row.

Belger, A., & Dichter, G. (2006). Structural and functional neuroanatomy. In J. A. Leberman, T. S. Stroup, & D. O. Perkins (Eds.), *The American psychiatric publishing textbook of schizophrenia* (pp. 167–185). Washington, DC: American Psychiatric Publishing.

Berry, J. W., & Kim, U. (1988). Accuration and mental health. In J. W. Dasen, J. W. Berry, & N. Sartorius (Eds.), *Health and cross-cultural psychology: Towards applications* (pp. 207—236). Thousand Oaks, CA: Sage.

Chambless, D. L., & Hollon, S. D. (1998). Defining empirically supported therapies. *Journal of Consulting and Clinical Psychology, 66,* 7–18.

Chambless, D. L., Sanderson, W. C., Shoham, V., Bennett Johnson, S., Pope, K. S., Crits-Christoph, P., Baker, M., Johnson, B., Woody, S. R., Sue, S., Beutler, L., Williams, D. A., & McCurry, S. (1996). An update on empirically validated therapies. *The Clinical Psychologist, 49,* 5–18.

Cheung, F. (1995). Facts and myths about somatization among the Chinese. In T. Y. Lin, W. S. Tseng, & E. K. Yeh (Eds.), *Chinese societies and mental health* (pp. 141–180). Hong Kong: Oxford University Press.

Constantine, M. G., Miville, M. L., Kindaichi, M. M., & Owens, D. (2010). Case conceptualizations of mental health counselors: Implications for the delivery of culturally competent care. In M. M. Leach, & J. D. Aten (Eds.), *Culture and the Therapeutic Process: A Guide for Mental Health Professionals* (pp. 99–115). New York, NY: Routledge.

Hardy, K. V., & Laszloffy, T. A. (2008). The dynamics of pro-racist ideology: Implications for family therapists. In M. McGoldrick & K. V. Hardy (Eds.), *Re-visioning family therapy: Race, culture, and gender in clinical practice* (pp. 225–249). New York, NY: Guildford Press.

Hinton, D. E., Chau, H., Nguyen, L., Nguyen, M., Pham, T., Quinn, S., & Tran, M. (2001). Panic disorder among Vietnamese refugees attending a psychiatric clinic: Prevalence and subtypes. *General Hospital Psychiatry, 23,* 337–344.

Hwang, W. (2007). Qi-gong psychotic reaction in a Chinese-American woman. *Culture, Medicine and Psychiatry, 31,* 547–560.

Hwang, W., Miranda, J., & Chung, C. (2007). Psychosis and shamanism in a Filipino-American immigrant. *Culture, Medicine and Psychiatry, 31,* 251–269.

Inman, A. G., Yeh, C. J., Madan-Bahel, A., & Nath, S. (2007). Bereavement and coping of South Asian families post 9/11. *Journal of Multicultural Counseling and Development, 35,* 101–115.

Kapur, S., & Lecrubier, I. (Eds.). (2003). *Dopamine in the pathophysiology and treatment of schizophrenia: New findings.* London, UK: Taylor & Francis.

Kingdon, D. G., & Turkington, D. (2005). *Cognitive therapy of schizophrenia: Guides to evidence-based practice.* New York, NY: Guilford.

Kinzie, J. D., Boehnlein, J. K., Leung, P. K., Moore, L. J., Riley, C., & Smith, D. (1990). The prevalence of posttraumatic stress disorder and its clinical significance among Southeast Asian refugees. *American Journal of Psychiatry, 147,* 913–917.

Ladany, N., Inman, A. G., Constantine, M. G., & Hofheinez, E. W. (1997). Supervisee multicultural case conceptualization ability and self-reported multicultural competence as functions of supervisee racial identity and supervisor focus. *Journal of Counseling Psychology, 44,* 284–293. doi: 10.1037/0022-0167.44.3.284

Leong, F. T. L., Leach, M., Yeh, C. J., & Chou, E. (2007). Suicide among Asian Americans: What do we know? What do we need to know? *Death Studies, 31*(5), 417–434. doi:10.1080/07481180701244561

Leong, F. T. L., & Lee, S. H. (2006). A cultural accommodation model of psychotherapy: Illustrated with the case of Asian-Americans. *Psychotherapy: Theory, Research, Practice, and Training, 43,* 410–423.

Phillips, L. J., Francey, S. M., Edwards, J., & McMurray, N. (2007). Stress and psychosis: Towards the development of new models of investigation. *Clinical Psychology Review, 27,* 307–317.

Rhee, S. (2009). The impact of immigration and acculturation on the mental health of Asian Americans: Overview of epidemiology and clinical implications. In N. H. Trinh, Y. Rho, F. Lu, & K. M. Sanders (Eds.). *Handbook of mental health and acculturation in Asian-American families* (pp. 81–98). New York, NY: Humana Press.

Sanchez, F., & Gaw, A. (2007). Mental health care of Filipino Americans. *Psychiatric Services, 58,* 810–815.

Shea, M., Yang, L. H., & Leong, F. T. L. (2010). Loss, psychosis, and chronic suicidality in a Korean-American immigrant man: Integration of cultural formulation model and multicultural case conceptualization. *Asian-American Journal of Psychology, 1,* 212–223.

Shen, B. J., & Takeuchi, D. T. (2001). A structural model of acculturation and mental health status among Chinese Americans. *American Journal of Community Psychology, 29,* 387–418.

Sue, D. W., & Sue, D. (2008). *Counseling the culturally diverse: Theory and practice* (5th Ed). Hoboken, NJ: Wiley.

Sullivan, H. S. (1962). *Schizophrenia as a human process.* New York, NY: Norton.

Tran, T. V. (1993). Psychological traumas and depression in a sample of Vietnamese people in the United States. *Health and Social Work, 18,* 184–94.

Tsuang, M. R., Stone, W. S., & Farone, S. V. (1999). Schizophrenia: A review of genetic studies. *Harvard Review of Psychiatry, 7,* 185–207.

Turkington, D., Kingdon, D., & Weiden, P. J. (2006). Cognitive behavioral therapy for schizophrenia. *American Journal of Psychiatry, 163,* 365–373

Yang, L. H., & Wonpat-Borja, A. (2006). Psychopathology among Asian Americans. In F. T. L. Leong, A. G. Inman, A. Elbreo, L. H. Yang, L. Kinoshita, & M. Fu (Eds.), *Handbook of Asian-American psychology* (2nd ed., pp. 379–404). Thousand Oaks, CA: Sage.

Concluding Remarks

What Can We Learn From Mental Health Practitioners Around the World?

Chalmer E. Thompson
Senel Poyrazli

We have much to learn from the contributors of this volume. But we begin with a look at the clients and patients first rather than the practitioners, as the accounts of these individuals can reveal much about the relationship. From the start of their contact with the practitioners to the end, these individuals were awakened to the possibility that they could discover better ways to cope and to feel more whole than when they first encountered these professionals. They practiced new ways of being in the world, found relief from the distress and trauma that plagued their lives, and improved their relationships with their children and parents. They stayed on with the relationship, experienced the struggle of seeming rejection by the therapist (e.g., Young Soon from Korea), encountered struggles that brought on further problems (e.g., Margaret Rukuni from Zimbabwe), and received encouragement to express themselves and behave in ways that departed from tradition, especially among the women clients (e.g., client JeeYoun from Korea and Mona from Lebanon). In Consoli, a los Ángeles Hernández Tzaquitzal, and González's chapter, the practitioners talked of the elicitation of *solidaridad*—mutual collaboration and commitment when faced with difficult, challenging, or painful situations; and *personalismo*—to treat one another with appreciation, consideration, and respect—born out of a view of one another as "you are I and I am you." Rukuni speaks of *ubuntu* which appears to have a similar meaning to Consoli et al.'s *personalismo,* and pertaining to the idea of one's own humanity as being wrapped up in another's humanity. In Gerstein, Kim, and Kim's chapter, a similar concept is conveyed in Han ideology with the lack of separation between the therapist and client. These concepts inform the practices of these professionals and there is evidence that these clients were in synch with them ideologically.

To us, that these people received the help they needed is a call to celebrate the maturity of a global mental health profession.

Also noteworthy is that the stigma in seeking help was perhaps lessened by the reputation of several practitioners. Regard had already been accorded María de los Ángeles Hernández Tzaquitzal in Guatemala, Young Soon Kim in Korea, and Mehmet Eskin in Turkey, as examples, likely making the decision for people in their communities to seek out the practitioner less of a challenge. Their exemplary practices stood out and the people showed that they were honored to know them and optimism about the care they would receive.

What we hope is also strongly evident in these pages is that culture is not fragile. It cannot be nor should not be ignored in the work of assessing individual or family problems, intervening with the people who need our help, and evaluating to determine if what we do is working. Culture is maintained despite people's transitions to new lands, as in the case of Mr. P. and Dr. Shea's personal accounts of migrating from China to the United States. Likewise, communities ruptured from natural disasters, civil wars and internments, and the spread of disease pose challenges to the unfurling of cultural learning, yet adults shore up their culturally based ways of coping for themselves and their children. In juxtaposition with modernity and hegemonic influences both within and outside of nations, culture both yields and resists simultaneously. Because of its utter complexity, there is the need for a stage on which culture can be understood, where people as cultural beings can be aptly described, and where healers can seriously contemplate how best to resolve the inevitable problems that surface when people experience distress in their lives.

What we illustrate in this volume is a glimpse of the stage on which their interventions take shape and some clues as to why these practitioners have been successful in building up the reputation of the profession in all corners of the world. The contributors to this volume are a sample of the best of what the mental health profession offers its local public because what these clients found was a professional who was able to capably understand them and caringly attend to their needs, or as Yujia Lei of China put it, who could lead them like "a guide that travels along on a journey."

In each and every one of the cases, the practitioner was perfectly clear about the value they place on their relationship with their clients or patients. As Valach and Young stated, "We addressed establishing the working alliance and relationship as the first issue in the client-counselor/psychotherapist encounter and it remains the highest priority throughout therapy." In other cases, the quality of the relationship comes across in the authors' description of the care and attention that is paid to the initial phases of the therapy (e.g., Guatemalan chapter). Intriguingly, although the theoretical tenets of U.S. theorist Carl Rogers's treatment model is mentioned in many of the chapters (i.e., providing empathy, being genuine and congruent, and providing unconditional acceptance as a way to build rapport and facilitate growth), in none of these instances are the facilitative conditions considered as sufficient to treatment success as Rogers proposed. Most authors emphasize the importance of establishing a sense of rapport and trust, especially in those cases where counseling and psychotherapy are new or when many people view these practices as stigmatizing.

Mental health practitioners in all of our chapters display how multicultural competency can be established in working with different people seeking help. As often discussed in the literature, a practitioner starts to become more culturally competent when he or she moves from being "culturally unaware to being aware . . . and to valuing and respecting differences" (Sue, Arredondo, & McDavis, 1992, p. 482). In addition, it is important to interview, design a treatment plan, and deliver psychological services based on client or patient characteristics, such as his or her sexual orientation, religious belief system, gender, age, socioeconomic background, or race-ethnicity (Hays, 2007). The practitioners in our book illustrate how they paid attention to these characteristics in their clients or patients. We also see that our practitioners paid attention to their own backgrounds (e.g., their gender, age, race-ethnicity, etc.) and how their backgrounds may have affected their dyadic relationships and also the treatment they provided. For example, Dr. Eskin discussed how being a heterosexual clinician who was supportive of lesbian, gay, bisexual, and transgendered (LGBT) rights contributed to his Turkish bisexual client's self-acceptance.

Spiritual aspects of the chapters were most evident in Roysircar's chapter (Haiti) as well as the chapters from the United States (Washington, DC), United States-China (Chinese-Immigrant), Guatemala, Lebanon, and Sierra Leone. These practitioners were able to understand and incorporate these spiritual aspects into the treatment, illustrating an aspect of the client or patient's being that is not conventionally addressed in Western literature. For practitioners like María de los Ángeles Hernández Tzaquitzal, this integration is part and parcel of their practice: According to Consoli et al., de los Ángeles Hernández Tzaquitzal "has been working on honing in an integrative perspective that organically brings together the Western ways of counseling and psychotherapy with the traditional ways of the Mayan cosmovision as narrated in the Popol Vuh, the sacred book of the K'iche' Maya people, *curanderismo* or indigenous healing, Catholic customs, and contemporary, alternative-healing methods."

The cultural accommodation model (CAM) presented by Shea and Leong offers practitioners a means to integrate cultural and sociopolitical influences into practice. For Shea, the revelation of her development as a practitioner is important to the chapter as many practitioners before her have and likely will continue to contemplate how they fit together traditional theories with life experiences that defy or question their application to all people. In the Shea and Leong chapter, Shea states, "The training in psychodynamic and cognitive-behavioral therapy (CBT) approaches has given me a breadth and depth of knowledge, strategies, and techniques to apply during the treatment process. The multicultural and postmodernist perspectives challenge me to consider my position and relation to my clients and how my clients and I construct the meaning of therapy together. I have learned to allow room for clients to tell their stories so I can understand problems and challenges from their perspectives. Rather than merely applying diagnostic labels and implementing treatment without cultural accommodation, I believe that it is important to understand the deeper meaning of clients' psychological problems, distress, functioning (whether adaptive or maladaptive), and indigenous coping within their sociocultural contexts." Shea mentions that she is humble in learning about her patient, even though the two share some commonalities. Humility is a word that comes to mind in our reading of Roysircar's chapter on the treatment of a Haitian family following the catastrophic January 12th earthquake.

A major thrust in preparing this volume was to identify international scholars and ask them to identify practitioners they knew who were well-known in their countries. In selecting these colleagues, all of whom we met in the United States, we took care to consider their dedication and talent. We chose the persons we believed to be some of the very best among the international psychologists we knew from our many years of involvement in the American Psychological Association (APA). These are scholars whose original homes were in countries other than the ones they currently reside, or who have studied and worked in more than one nation. In our minds, their scholarship emulated worldliness and sensitivity in the peoples of the world. We have come to respect them, knew that they passed on their knowledge to students and colleagues alike, and when we asked that they again share their wisdom to new readers, they heeded our calls. And of our practitioners, we found what we were looking for: caring and competent professionals who wanted first and foremost to know their helpees well and to gain their trust in what they do.

Earlier as noted, our selection of scholars was composed of colleagues we met in the United States. We limited ourselves to those whose associations crossnationally were tied to others who were trained using Western models of therapy. Consequently, we were not surprised that most of the practitioners had been influenced by these models. For example, in Duan et al., the authors make liberal use of two theories that can be seen by many as having incompatible aims: Rogerian and insight-oriented therapies. They make use of the psychodynamics theories, ever mindful of the pathological leanings of the language (e.g., weak ego strength) but keep a steady focus on the client growth and the here-and-now. Their departure from this primarily here-and-now approach is seen in the provision of insight to the client but not the sort of insight related to family dynamics and intrapsychic conflicts. Instead, the therapist attends to the contextual forces that obstruct his ability to function optimally and feel worthy as a human being. The authors address the pressures that can occur for young people in Chinese society when the competition for highly prized placements at universities is stiff. Being every mindful of the need to bring honor to the family combined with cultural values that suppress outward revealing about parental weakness or shortcomings, the counselor shows her regard for her client as she focuses attention on the cultural context and talks of her admiration of the client.

Departures from Westernized therapies were also observed. Brigitte Khoury spoke definitively of the salience of family members taking part in psychotherapy as the family becomes "one of the most important allies in treatment." Although family systems theorists from the United States and Europe address this salience, Khoury's treatise about the family's role shows regard for the curiosities—indeed, suspicions, that occur when the individual is in treatment and the need for parents to assume their rightful positions culturally in knowing what the therapy is about and how it is proceeding. Khoury's chapter beautifully illustrates how some of the intrusions of family can be incorporated into this respect for family and balanced with the wishes of her patient to have a less-obtrusive life with her husband and son while affirming her love and respect for her parents.

As Cushman (1995) noted in his statement that psychotherapy occurs within context and is therefore never universal, these practitioners reveal to us that they take into account matters of modernity as they necessarily and wisely contemplate the integration of approaches that are Western-based and indigenous to the region. When the helpee receives help from a country outside the one in which he was reared, as in the case of Mr. P from Vietnam, the practitioner needs to avail him or herself of the cultural resources that can best help the client while determining ways to inform him of new cultural practices. Questions like "How does an increasing proclivity toward individuality (over collectivism) influence my work with youthful clients?" are the sort that have to be contemplated as the professional sets forth the essential goal of knowing his helpee.

Another emergent feature in these chapters is that people all over the world differ in terms of the availability or access to mental health care in their respective communities or societies. In Switzerland, for example, universal health care exists. As a result, individuals wanting to receive psychological treatment are provided extensive coverage that allows utilization of different treatment approaches and provides the opportunity to treat cases requiring long-term therapy. As another example, we read that in Turkey, a non-Western country, mental health treatment is treated at the same level as physical health treatment in that clients and patients can see a psychiatrist or a psychologist as many times as they like. In addition, their visits are covered by their insurance. Despite the positive side of insurance coverage, we also would like to point out that in some of these communities finding a professional seems to be a challenge due to having a smaller number of mental health practitioners in comparison to the need in the community. Moreover, on college campuses in Korea and China, counseling centers are flourishing, as indicated in the chapters by Duan et al. and Gerstein et al. The cost of these services is absorbed in students' fees.

In far too many countries, the availability of mental health practitioners is limited, as pointed out in the chapters by Roysircar on her work in Haiti, and by Kalayjian and Sofletea in Sierra Leone. Abject poverty, combined with the ravages of war, the spread of disease, and the crimes that are an outgrowth of a disintegration of communities and tribes that arise from these formative ills, far too frequently translates into an absence of professional care of any sort, and this matter of such meager resources available to some while others are swollen with wealth, is a reality that bears reckoning. In cases from all over the world, mental health practitioners who deliver only counseling and psychotherapy are a luxury. And from what we have read in our crisis cases, the expanded offer of services is essential to the lives of those they service.

Four of the chapters in the volume address people whose regions are populated mostly by African-descended people, specifically Haiti, Sierra Leone, the United States (Washington, DC), and Zimbabwe. In all but one of the chapters, the interventions are crisis related. The exception is in the U.S. case where the client was relatively (presumably) wealthy. This issue of economics figures prominently in our display of cases around the world.

We were strongly motivated to select chapters not only from developing countries but also from those regions of the world where there ostensibly are recorded accounts of economic, social, and political progress in addition to seemingly intractable challenges. We believed strongly that our volume would not be quite complete without addressing the experiences of those whose lives are affected by the onslaught of the world's disasters, natural or human-made, and combined; and in the cases of these nations, the impacts of prolonged exposure to poverty and oppression on the well-being of a people.

Andrew Mwenda (Mwenda, 2007) talks about the need of Western media to refrain from devoting most of their attention to negative aspects of Africa and hence, concentrating on poverty and despair, rather than the strengths and potential that exist on the massive continent. The reframing should be one of moving from a poverty reduction need to one of creating wealth. Sending charity for the hungry or peace-keepers to the countries that experience civil wars, as Mwenda notes, are efforts to treat the symptoms, not the causes of Africa's fundamental problems. As the editors of this book, we make the same appeal to those growing numbers of professionals who see a need to reduce the incidences of psychological despair in Africa and other developing countries already strapped with serious problems. There is no question that the despair ought to be erased, just as poverty needs to be reduced. Creating wealth in psychological terms is to advance partnerships that will foster the establishment of mental health as a fixture in these societies.

Reporting on the impacts of some sociopolitical factors is controversial and it is not uncommon that many practitioners around the world may hesitate to discuss these factors in writing, fearing possible repercussions. In some of the chapters, especially in societies where speaking openly is an aspiration, we see lengthy discussions of sociopolitical contexts and their impact on the person receiving help. In some other chapters, however, many authors could not discuss these contexts freely in writing, while we knew from our private communications with them that they were fully aware of the impact these contexts had on the individuals.

Finally, we want to conclude that this book could be taken as merely more of the same: pandering to the notion that psychological problems are treated and people then merely return to living their lives, many of whom experience considerable torment and oppression because of societal forces that impose dehumanizing messages about the worth of a people based on their race or ethnicity, religion, economic standing, and sexual orientation. Do mental health practitioners continue to try fixing problems that are outgrowths of sick societies (Smith, 1985) or do we broaden our skills as Rukuni, Kalayjian and Sofletea, and Roysircar do, or infuse approaches that attune to the more systemic ills as with Shea and Leong?

Psychology training programs that incorporate social justice approaches are needed as in the programs at Boston College (see Goodman et al., 2004) and at the Ball State University as described in this volume by Gerstein, Kim, and Kim. And as Watts (2004) points out, future developments of social justice–oriented programs need to take deliberate efforts to enfold people from *all* backgrounds, thereby overcoming the structural issues that keep certain people in and others out.

We offer a final challenge to readers as we reflect on the harrowing descriptions by Rukuni and Roysircar of what the people of Zimbabwe and Haiti experience. As there are increases in the numbers of psychologists partnering across nations, we must deliberately and creatively disrupt patterns of relating by breaking down structural barriers to genuine collaboration. Wealthy nations remain wealthy and even become wealthier, while the poorest of our nations seem intractably caught up in poverty. The multiculturalism literature is swollen with research studies and theories that provide useful tools for creating needed change at different ecological levels and the need for scaling up these tools to apply to cross-national activities among psychologists is ever so ripe. We have to first believe, as former United Nations secretary Kofi Annan (2006), once stated, that global solidarity is not only necessary but also possible. Annan states further that

it is necessary because without a measure of solidarity, no society can be truly stable, and no one's prosperity truly secure. That applies to national societies—as all the great industrial democracies learned in the 20th century—but it also applies to the increasingly integrated global market economy we live in today. It is not realistic to think that some people can go on deriving great benefits from globalization while billions of their fellow human beings are left in abject poverty or even thrown into it. We have to give our fellow citizens, not only within each nation but in the global community, at least a chance to share in our prosperity.

When we are able to share in our prosperity as mental health practitioners and scholars, then we will have achieved the pinnacle of internationalization. But there is much work in reaching this goal. In our strivings, we need to continue summoning the knowledge of scholars and practitioners from developing countries and make every effort to create collaborations in which these perspectives are not merely included but also deemed equally as relevant and not marginalized. During our strivings we will surely wrangle, grapple, and disagree with another practitioner's perspective on forgiveness, for example, or on the use of therapy as a social justice tool. These disagreements are essential to our learning, and rather than turn away from one another in discord, we need to continue our march toward the goal of ensuring that people who need our help derive the fullest of benefits of our struggle. Ultimately, we want to ensure that there is regard for all humanity, as conveyed in the words of our contributors who speak of the humanity of each one of us as being wrapped up in the humanity in one another.

References

Annan, K. (2006, December 11). Secretary-General Kofi Annan's address at the Truman Presidential Museum & Library. Retrieved from http://www.un.org/apps/sg/sgstats.asp?nid=2357

Cushman, P. (1995). *Constructing the self, constructing America: A cultural history of psychotherapy*. New York, NY: Addison-Wesley.

Goodman, L. A., Liang, E., Helms, J. E., Latta, R. E., Sparks, E., Weintraub, S. R. (2004). Training counseling psychologists as social justice agents: Feminist and multicultural principles in action. *The Counseling Psychologist, 32*, 793–837.

Hays, P. A. (2007). *Addressing cultural complexities in practice, assessment, diagnosis, and therapy*. Washington, DC: American Psychological Association.

Mwenda, Andrew. (2007, September). Andrew Mwenda takes a new look at Africa [Video file]. Retrieved from http://www.ted.com/talks/lang/eng/andrew_mwenda_takes_a_new_look_at_africa.html

Smith, E. M. J. (1985). Ethnic minorities: Life stress, social support, and mental health issues. *The Counseling Psychologist, 13*, 537–579.

Sue, D. W., Arredondo, P., & McDavis, R. J. (1992). Multicultural counseling competencies and standards: A call to the profession. *Journal of Counseling and Development, 70*, 477–486.

Watts, R. (2004). Integrating social justice and psychology. *The Counseling Psychologist, 32*, 855–865.

Index _____

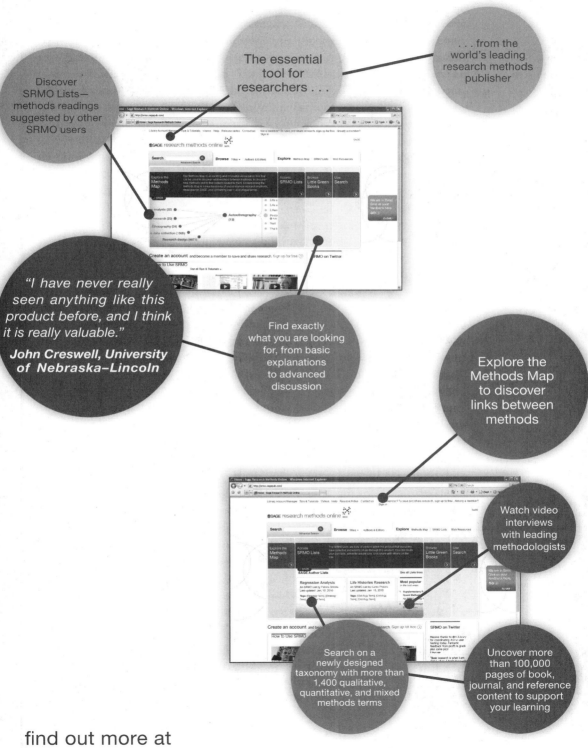

SAGE research**methods**
The Essential Online Tool for Researchers

. . . from the world's leading research methods publisher

The essential tool for researchers . . .

Discover SRMO Lists—methods readings suggested by other SRMO users

"*I have never really seen anything like this product before, and I think it is really valuable.*"

John Creswell, University of Nebraska–Lincoln

Find exactly what you are looking for, from basic explanations to advanced discussion

Explore the Methods Map to discover links between methods

Watch video interviews with leading methodologists

Search on a newly designed taxonomy with more than 1,400 qualitative, quantitative, and mixed methods terms

Uncover more than 100,000 pages of book, journal, and reference content to support your learning

find out more at
srmo.sagepub.com